Your Cleft-Affected Child

DEDICATION

"A Journey of a thousand miles must begin with a single step."
—Lao-Tzu, Tao Te Ching

"The distance is nothing. It's only the first step that's important."
—Marquise du Deffand (1763)

To my Aiden, whose courage in the face of pain and perseverance
in the smallest of successes has made him my hero.
And to my older children, all of whom have loved and helped
Aiden every step of the way: Kaitlynne, Aaron, Alex, and Kelsey.
Your sacrifices have not gone unnoticed.

Ordering

Trade bookstores in the U.S. and Canada please contact:

Publishers Group West
1700 Fourth Street, Berkeley CA 94710
Phone: (800) 788-3123   Fax: (800) 351-5073

Hunter House books are available at bulk discounts for textbook course adoptions; to qualifying community, health care, and government organizations; and for special promotions and fund-raising. For details please contact:

Special Sales Department
Hunter House Inc., PO Box 2914, Alameda CA 94501-0914
Phone: (510) 865-5282   Fax: (510) 865-4295
E-mail: ordering@hunterhouse.com

Individuals can order our books from most bookstores,
by calling **(800) 266-5592,**
or from our website at **www.hunterhouse.com**

Your Cleft- Affected Child

The Complete Book of Information, Resources, and Hope

CARRIE T. GRUMAN-TRINKNER

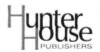
Hunter House
PUBLISHERS

Hunter House Inc., Publishers
PO Box 2914
Alameda CA 94501-0914

Library of Congress Cataloging-in-Publication Data

Gruman-Trinkner, Carrie T.
Your cleft-affected child: the complete book of information, resources, and hope / Carrie Gruman-Trinkner. — 1st ed.
p. cm.
ISBN-13: 978-0-89793-185-4 (pb) — ISBN-10: 0-89793-185-8 (pb)
1. Cleft palate children. 2. Cleft palate. 3. Cleft lip. I. Title.
RD525 .G78 2001
618.92'0975225—dc21   2001026471

Project Credits

Cover Design: Peri Poloni, Knockout Design
Illustrator: Marty J. Granius
Book Production: Hunter House
Copy Editor: Bevin McLaughlin
Proofreader: Lee Rappold
Indexer: Kathy Talley-Jones
Acquisitions Editor: Jeanne Brondino
Associate Editor: Alexandra Mummery
Editorial and Production Assistant: Emily Tryer
Acquisitions and Publicity Assistant: Lori Covington
Sales and Marketing Assistant: Earlita K. Chenault
Publicity Manager: Sara Long
Customer Service Manager: Christina Sverdrup
Order Fulfillment: Joel Irons
Administrator: Theresa Nelson
Computer Support: Peter Eichelberger
Publisher: Kiran S. Rana

Manufactured in the United States of America

9 8 7 6 5 4 3 2   First Edition   10 11 12 13 14

Contents

Important Note

The material in this book is intended to provide a review of resources and information related to cleft disorders. Every effort has been made to provide accurate and dependable information. However, professionals in the field may have differing opinions and change is always taking place. Any of the treatments described herein should be undertaken only under the guidance of a licensed health care practitioner. The author, editors, and publishers cannot be held responsible for any error, omission, professional disagreement, outdated material, or adverse outcomes that derive from use of any of these treatments or information resources in this book, either in a program of self-care or under the care of a licensed practitioner.

Foreword

It's been almost 40 years since I was born with a cleft lip and palate, and I must say it has been some ride—a ride that has made me thankful it happened. It has at times been tough, but boy, what a blessing it's been in the long run. My birth defect has caused me to spend less time worried about the things most people worry about most of the time. It has helped me focus on taking action.

While so many people define themselves by words, I learned to define myself by the things I did. (It's funny to think that now I speak for a living.) Because of my birth defect, I have learned to see the world and judge the world differently. I have learned to see beauty in what others consider ugly. Despite—or because of—the challenges put to me by others' behavior, I have learned that none of us is flawless, and that the way to peace is through love.

To those who have a child with a cleft: realize your actions speak volumes. The love my family showed me as a child helped me realize the value of my being born different. They handled all those things that came with my cleft as challenges that would create character and add depth to my personality. This goes out to all of you who either have a cleft-affected child or know someone who has a cleft or a cleft-affected child. Today may be hard, but, as in all things, the best comes to those who can persevere. May this book give you the vision needed to see what I know to be true: that being born with a cleft is not a burden, but a defining mark of worth.

> — **Blaise Winter,** a cleft-affected child, a college graduate, a professional athlete, a husband, a father, a professional speaker, an author, and a happy man.

Born with a unilateral cleft lip and palate, Winter faced adversity at a young age. After discovering his talent at football, Winter found the acceptance he had always craved. Playing for the Indianapolis Colts, Winter was named to the NFL's First Team All-Rookie list. He continued in the NFL, playing for the Green Bay Packers and the San Diego Chargers. He ended his career with a damaged knee, standing on the sidelines as his team vied for a Super Bowl Championship. (They lost to the San Francisco 49ers.) Winter's first book, A Reason to Believe, describes growing up with a cleft palate and his experiences in the NFL. Winter is now a motivational speaker whose work has brought hope to thousands of people.

Acknowledgments

There are many people who have helped in the formation of this book: nurses, physicians, therapists, parents of cleft-affected children, cleft-affected adults and teens, and the little ones who speak so easily of their situations. I have found that the people of the cleft-affected community are incredibly open, ready to share personal experience and insight if it will help others in any way.

Thank you to Kaitlynne, Aaron, Alex, Kelsey, and Aiden who had to "give up Momma time" every once in a while, but could always be counted on for a snuggle at the right moment. My gratitude to Jenny Westenberger, Michelle VandeYacht, Melanie Horn, Kara Delzer, Lucia Moberg, Christian Smith, and Mary Sanders, whose time with my children freed me to help others.

To Marty J. Granius, Justin Woods, Theresa Thomas, Blaise Winter, and those anonymous friends whose belief in this work, and contributions to it, will help so many others.

Thank you to Max Lippert, Amara Rose DeLaruelle, Brian Price, Jan Johnston, Ed Berthiaume, Tom Richards, Cyndi Vander Pas, Dawn Trettin-Moyer, Jeanne Juve, Deacon Vin De Groot; to Marshall Cooke, Christine DeSmet, Sabra Steimke for their enthusiasm and help over the years; to Heidi Teal for her love and help in Aiden's early years, as well as for being a fount of information for this book; to Lynn Goldapske for the miracles wrought in Aiden's speech; to Dr. Kurt Heyrman and Dr. Mark Faustich; to Dr. Steven Hardy and all of the men and women on the team at the University of Wisconsin Hospitals in Madison; and to Mike Rietveld and my colleagues in the Kimberly School District for their help and understanding with both Aiden's procedures and the publication of this book. Thank you to Jennifer

Siebers, whose encouragement and help have given my family a new lease on life. You will be deeply missed.

Thank you to my agent, Scott Edelstein, and my editors, Jeanne Brondino, Alexandra Mummery, and Bevin McLaughlin, at Hunter House—your patience and advice have been invaluable. Thank you for your understanding in the midst of great personal tragedy.

To Debbie Sonnleitner for her patience and invaluable help!

To my precious family: Tom and Eileen Gruman, Mark and Katie Gruman, Bernadette Gruman Shirley, Mary and Craig Ellenbecker, Sherry Gruman, Tommy, Mari, Sarah, Jake, Megan, Emily, Taylor, and Madi. Your love and support have given Aiden such a bright beginning, and your belief in my work has been a lifeline.

And to my beloved brother Ray, whose belief in me is the greatest gift he could have given. I will miss our long talks and your ready laugh as I told you stories of Aiden's successes. I will never forget your comforting hugs, an arm slung around my shoulders, and assurances that "It'll be okay. Aiden will be just fine." I always called you before each surgery because you told me Aiden would be okay. I believed you then, and I believe you even more now that you are in heaven watching over him.

INTRODUCTION

A Beacon of Hope

Congratulations on the birth of your baby! There is nothing quite like the sweet smell of an infant, the feel of her soft skin snuggling up against you, the tickle of her warm breath on your neck. However, not every aspect of this new birth has brought you joy. Right now you are probably experiencing a confusing mixture of emotions: happiness, relief, shock, fear, anger, and perhaps even guilt. Your baby was born with a cleft, and you might not be fully prepared to deal with this facial difference and the emotions it generates. I know exactly where you are, because not long ago I was there, too. My own son was born with a complete bilateral cleft of his lip, gum, and palate. Please know that you are not alone—and you have every reason for hope and optimism.

First, let me assure you emphatically that *this is not your fault.* No matter what anyone tells you, believe the truth of that statement. There is no evidence in any study that shows a clear cause-and-effect association between clefting and factors such as the mother's nutrition, exercise, alcohol or drug use, or emotions.

You may feel like you are alone in the challenging and often terrifying position of having a child with a cleft lip or palate. However, as you become more aware of clefting and begin to recognize its effects, you may begin to notice many people in your community who were born with clefts. In fact, with the birth incidence of clefting so high (1 in 700 births on average), there are a lot more cleft-affected people in the world than you may realize. This book is designed to show you that you are not alone on your path. As proof that your child does not need to see a cleft lip or palate as a stumbling block, throughout the book you will find bios of famous athletes, actors, and others who were born with clefts themselves or who are raising children who were born with clefts.

This book is meant as a beacon of hope. Between these covers you will find all the information you need on clefting, its causes, and its treatment. A wealth of information on a variety of associated issues, such as hearing, speech, and dental and orthodontic work, will be offered.

In addition, you'll find assistance and support in dealing with the emotional effects of clefting on your child and your family, as well as tips on dealing with the reactions of others. Along the way, this book will provide you with information on financial matters; an education packet to be shared with elementary school classmates; speech charts; information on forming a support or advocacy group; a list of additional resources; and a glossary defining the often difficult terminology associated with clefting and its treatment.

Lastly, *Your Cleft-Affected Child* will provide you with encouragement and inspiration through the stories of many successful people who were born with clefts. Accompanying photographs will provide absolute proof that your child has every hope of having a beautiful, whole face with minimal (or completely invisible) scarring. Within these pages, you will find the answers to your questions and concerns. More important, you will find hope and empowerment. You will learn how to become your child's greatest asset in his recovery. In the process, your own fear, worry, and confusion will ease as well. Turn the page, and together let's begin to build new hope for your precious child.

CHAPTER 1

Types of Clefts and Their Causes

What Is a Cleft?

Here is the single most important thing you need to know about clefting: it is normally fully correctable through surgery, with minimal scarring. The result is generally 100 percent normal functioning—and, usually, a completely normal appearance as well. In short, with surgery, your child should be just fine. Nevertheless, the appearance of a cleft lip can be startling. If you are concerned that the cleft causes some physical pain in your baby, don't be. Clefting is not an injury. Your baby is not in pain.

A cleft is a *congenital birth defect*. In other words, something occurred in the womb when your baby was forming that caused parts of his or her mouth to remain open and unconnected. The word *cleft* means "split" or "divided." When you look at your baby's cleft, the word will seem fitting. You'll see a split in the child's lip and/or roof of the mouth (the *palate*). The split may also appear in the upper gum (*alveolar ridge*). The term for a split in the lip is *cleft lip*; the term for a split in the roof of the mouth is *cleft palate*. In years past, a cleft was commonly called a *harelip*, due to a perceived resemblance to the split lip of a rabbit. This label is currently considered offensive, however, and is best avoided.

Clefting may occur in the lip, gum, or palate, or any combination of the three. It can happen on one side or on both sides. It can also, in more rare occasions, occur as a *midline* defect—a horseshoe-shaped palate cleft. A hidden, or *submucous*, cleft can also be present in the palate. A *complete cleft lip* extends into the nostrils. Similarly, a *complete cleft palate* extends the entire length of the roof of the mouth, from the back to the front. An *incomplete cleft* involves a smaller portion of the lip or palate. Cleft presentations are as individual as your child.

Unilateral Cleft

A cleft on one side is called a *unilateral cleft*. It may be present in varying degrees of severity, from a small notch at the edge of the lip to a complete separation from the nostril through the lip, gum, and palate. Children with a complete unilateral cleft lip will generally have a misshapen nose, with the *nasal ala* (the skin outside the nostril) on the clefted side being more flat and distended. Once your child's lip is repaired, the shape of the nose becomes

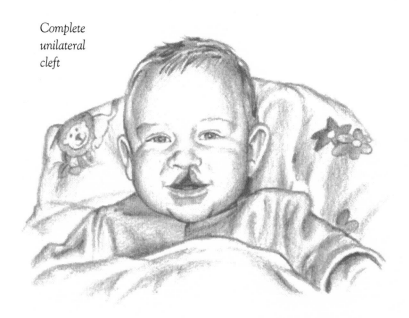

Complete unilateral cleft

Incomplete
unilateral
clefts

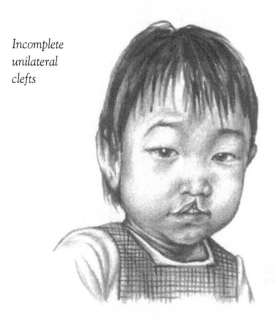

more normal. Sometimes nose revision surgery is necessary to complete the repair.

A unilateral cleft palate, likewise, is a split along one side of the roof of the mouth. A cleft palate may involve the *uvula* (the U-shaped piece of skin that hangs down from the palate into the throat) or it may be as simple as a small notch in the back of the

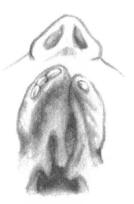

Complete cleft palate

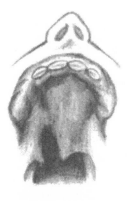

Incomplete cleft palate

soft palate, or *velum* (the soft portion of the roof of the mouth closest to the throat). Or it may be as severe as a cleft through both the soft and hard palate (the hard portion of the roof of the mouth closest to the front teeth). A unilateral cleft palate may appear alone or in conjunction with a cleft lip.

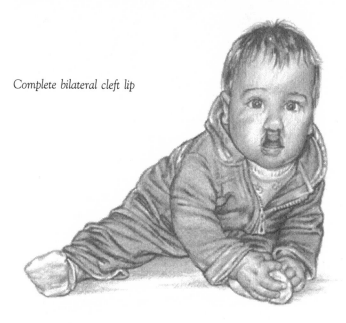

Complete bilateral cleft lip

Bilateral Cleft

If a cleft appears on both sides of the lip or palate, it is called a *bilateral cleft*. Like a unilateral cleft, the bilateral cleft can vary in degrees of severity. One side may be less severe than the other, or the two clefts may be identical. Generally, however, one cleft will appear wider than the other. This type of clefting may affect the lip, gum, or palate, or any combination of the three. A child with a severe bilateral cleft lip may have a portion of the gum protruding forward. This piece is called the *premaxilla*. It may resemble a little duckbill, or it may have collapsed inward. Generally, lip surgery can gently push the premaxilla into alignment. Further surgery can fuse the gum line.

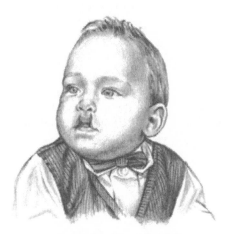

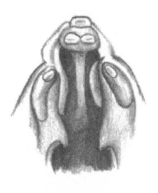

Incomplete bilateral cleft lip

Complete bilateral
cleft palate

The nose of a child with a bilateral cleft lip will have a tendency to flatten. The *columella* (the strip of skin between the nostrils) may not be of normal length. This, too, can be repaired in a standard surgical procedure.

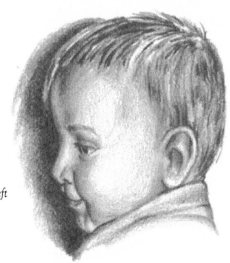

Profile of bilateral cleft
showing flat nose

A bilateral cleft palate involves both sides of the palate. A complete bilateral cleft palate will look as though the roof of the mouth is missing. It is not really missing, of course; it simply did not come together and fuse properly.

Submucous Cleft

A submucous cleft is often called a *hidden cleft* because it cannot be seen at birth. This type of cleft involves the muscles of the soft palate, but not the lining of the palate. Hence, the child will appear at first glance to have an intact palate. Because it is not immediately visible, a submucous cleft may be diagnosed later than an apparent cleft.

How a Cleft Forms

A baby's face begins to develop between the 4th and 8th weeks of pregnancy. The lip and palate form independently, with the lip forming first, followed by the palate a few weeks later. Actually, every one of us starts life in the womb with a cleft lip. However, in most people, the lip comes together and fuses, forming two lines below our nostrils called *philtral lines.* Likewise, the roof of everyone's mouth begins with a bilateral cleft; the palate then comes together and fuses. (You can feel and see the fusion "scars" below the nose and along the middle of the palate.) A congenital cleft occurs when, for some reason, fusion does not take place. In other words, a cleft lip or palate did not separate or split apart, but simply did not come together. A cleft is generally in place within the first 6 weeks of pregnancy, and often occurs before a woman is even aware of being pregnant.

Causes of Clefting

About one-third of all clefting is due to hereditary factors. Most clefts appear to occur at random, and studies have found no definitive cause of nonhereditary clefts. Theories about maternal factors involved in clefting include malnutrition, vitamin A (too lit-tle or too much), the use of certain drugs, and interrupted blood flow in the womb. None of these theories has been conclusively proven. In fact, there have been cases of identical twins (who share the same genetic makeup and, obviously, the same envi-ronment) of whom one has a cleft and the other does not.

It is possible that certain medications, illegal drugs, alcohol, or smoking may disrupt the development of a fetus at a critical stage. If this disruption occurs in the early weeks of pregnancy, birth defects—including clefting—may be more likely to occur (Evidence is still inconclusive, however.) A Boston University School of Medicine study has indicated that women who con-sume excessive amounts of vitamin A are more likely to have infants with malformations of the head, face, heart, and brain. Other theories point to obstructions as the cause of some clefts. For example, a baby may be curled tightly in the womb with his chin down. His tongue may be forced to remain up at the roof of the mouth, getting in the way of proper fusion. In the same way, a tiny fist or other body part may obstruct fusion. Some stud-ies have indicated that clefting is more likely to occur in twins and other multiple births than in single births.

One rare but documented cause of obstructional clefting is known as Constriction Band Syndrome. This condition can occur when, during early pregnancy, there is a rupture in the amniotic sac. Although this generally causes spontaneous abortion or mis-carriage, in certain incidences the baby continues to develop. Because there is no amniotic sac, the baby can become entan-gled in the *chorion*, filaments on the outer part of the placenta. The chorion can then constrict the growth of the body parts around which these filaments are tangled. Several results are pos-sible, including clubfeet, *syndactyly* (fusing or webbing of the fin-gers or toes), loss of a limb, or lack of growth of a limb. If the rupture in the amniotic sac occurs very early, clefting may result. Accidents in which either the amniotic sac or the placenta is damaged may also account for some cleft formations. (The acci-dent would have to occur within the first 2 months of pregnancy.)

Several tall tales still abound regarding the causes of non-hereditary clefting. One is that the fetus injured itself by thumb sucking or scratching its mouth with its fingernails. Another is that the mother was within close proximity to a rabbit during the first month of pregnancy. Both of these notions are pure myth, with absolutely no basis in fact.

Genetic Factors in Clefting

A *syndrome* is a group of symptoms or effects that are caused by a single factor. In the case of genetic syndromes, an abnormal gene will cause one or more developmental differences to occur. Several known syndromes may include clefting as one of their components. Parents who carry genes for these syndromes have a higher statistical chance of having a child with a cleft. For example, in the chart below, each parent carries a dominant (A) and a recessive (*a*) gene. The four possible combinations of the genes would be AA, A*a*, *a*A, and *aa*. If the recessive gene caused clefting, the *aa* combination of genes would result in a child with a cleft. These parents would therefore have a one-in-four likelihood of having a child with a cleft.

Mother		Father	
Aa		Aa	
Child 1	Child 2	Child 3	Child 4
AA	Aa	aA	aa

However, a parent with an *autosomal dominant* genetic condition, which requires only one dominant dysfunctional gene to be present in the child, has a fifty-fifty chance of passing on the condition. Van Der Voude Syndrome, for example, is an autosomal dominant genetic condition which can include a cleft lip, a cleft palate, or both, as well as missing teeth and lip pits. Stickler Syndrome is another autosomal dominant condition. Stickler can include progressive myopia, retinal detachment, hearing loss, clefting, joint pain, and other symptoms. Other genetically caused syndromes which can include clefting—but which are far less likely to be passed on than an autosomal dominant condition—are Arhinia, Hemifacial Microsomia (also called Goldenhar), Kallman Syndrome (which is often associated with median facial clefts), Oral Facial Digital Syndrome Type I (characterized by asymmetric and irregular clefts, as well as other physical malformations), Cornelia DeLange Syndrome, and some growth hormone deficiencies.

Parents have no control over their genetic make-up. Often they have no idea they carry a gene for one of these syndromes, since it is possible to do so yet not have that syndrome oneself. Determining that a syndromes or genetic cause is present requires that a geneticist make a firm diagnosis after testing the child, the parents, or both. Genetic testing may consist of a simple interview, lasting approximately 2 hours, during which family history and personal health issues are explored. Some genetic work may require a blood sample.

Pierre Robin Sequence

A *sequence*, as opposed to a syndrome, is similar to a domino effect. One factor causes another, which, in turn, triggers another factor. Pierre Robin Sequence is thought to originate with a small jaw, resulting in displacement of the tongue, which, in turn, impairs proper palate closure. Children with Robin's generally exhibit the following symptoms: *micrognathia* (an underdeveloped lower jaw), *glossoptosis* (a "floppy" tongue), a severely cleft palate (usually in a *U* shape), and associated breathing problems.

Don't Blame Yourself

Many a new mother of a cleft-affected child has needlessly tortured herself with guilt over the condition. However, since there are no definitive causes of clefting, it serves no purpose to assign blame to either parent, to the environment, or to the child. Take comfort in the fact that your baby's facial difference was caused by factors beyond your control. It is *not* your—nor anyone else's—fault. Sometimes a pregnancy is unplanned and, as a result, the mother may privately wish she were not pregnant. She may even wish for the baby to miscarry. She may be angry or depressed about having a child. *None of these emotions can cause a cleft.* In fact, in most cases, the cleft forms before the mother knows she is pregnant.

Other mothers may have hoped for a girl rather than a boy, or a boy rather than a girl. When a baby of the longed-for gender arrives with a cleft, the mother may believe she is being punished for not appreciating a baby of either gender. First, realize that a baby, any baby, is never a punishment. Second, know that wishes, hopes, and dreams are not wrong—and they will not result in a child with a facial difference. Maternal emotions, no matter how strong, cannot and do not cause clefts.

Some Helpful Numbers

About 1 child in 33 is born with some type of birth defect. The most common birth defects are heart and circulation defects (1 in 115 births), muscle and skeletal defects (1 in 130 births), and clefting, which affects about 1 in 700 children. Cleft lips, with or without an accompanying cleft palate, occur more often in boys than girls. Cleft palates alone are seen more frequently in girls. However, in general, clefting is 50 percent more common in boys than in girls. The likelihood of clefting varies among racial and ethnic groups, presumably because of genetic factors. The highest likelihood of clefting (1 in 500 births) occurs among Asian, Latin, and Native American groups. Children of European descent have clefts in 1 in 600 to 700 births. Blacks are the least likely to be born with clefts, with clefting occurring in 1 in 1,000 births.

Some concern has arisen in recent years over an apparent increase in the rate of some birth defects, including cleft lips and cleft palates. It must be noted, however, that medical advances, better prenatal care, and improved nutrition have lowered mortality rates for cleft-affected babies. This is certainly a factor in the higher occurrence of live births of babies with facial differences.

Stacy Keach, Actor and Director

One of the more famous cleft-affected celebrities, Stacy Keach has been an outspoken advocate for the cleft-affected community. The star of "Mike Hammer" and "Titus," Keach has had numerous other stage and film credits, including American History X. Born with a cleft lip and incomplete cleft palate, Mr. Keach had his first surgery at 6 months of age. He had four operations in all, which he describes as "traumatic." As a teenager, Keach opted against having further revisions. According to Keach, his cleft scar has never been an issue in his romantic life: "Women thought it was sexy, so that was good."

Passing It On

A parent with an autosomal dominant genetic condition has a 50 percent chance of passing on that condition to her child. Parents with recessive genes for certain genetic conditions have a one in four chance of having a child with a cleft. Only certain tests can truly determine the presence of a genetic condition. However, one must be aware that even these tests have a margin of error. One can question the geneticist about this likelihood at the time of testing. Genetic testing may include a history of cleft occurrences in your and your spouse's immediate and extended families, some simple blood tests, or cell scrapings for DNA. Of course, unless you have your genes tested—or you already know that clefting runs in your or your spouse's family—you cannot know whether such a risk is present. So let's look briefly at the more general statistics.

A father with a cleft (and with no family history of clefting) has a 5 percent chance of having a cleft-affected child. The same rate generally applies to the mother. If both parents of a child with a cleft have no history of clefting, there is a 1 in 25 chance of their having a second baby with a cleft. If a mother has a cleft and she has one child with a cleft, however, her odds of having a second cleft-affected child jump to 1 in 10. If you already have two or more children with clefts, each child born thereafter probably has at least a 25 percent chance of being born with a cleft as well. Almost certainly some genetic factors causing clefting are involved.

Some Final Words

As Joanne Green, mother (by adoption) of three cleft-affected children and founder of Wide Smiles, has put it: "Remember that the baby you hold is a baby first, and cleft-affected second." Of all the things you need to know about your child with facial differences, this is one of the most important. Now that we know what clefting is, how it occurs, and what causes it, let's look at what can be done to repair it.

CHAPTER 2

How Can This Be Fixed?

This chapter contains information intended to be used solely as an educational guide for parents on various options for their child's care. It is in no way intended to take the place of professional medical decisions. Each child's situation is unique and only the physicians attending that child are qualified to make the decisions appropriate for his unique cleft presentation. This chapter may be used as a stepping stone in a parent's basic knowledge of the team approach to cleft repair, surgery, and postsurgical care. Parents must seek professional advice before taking any action concerning the reconstruction of their child's cleft.

The Team Approach to Cleft Palate Care

Although there are plastic surgeons who work alone on children with cleft presentations, it is generally advisable to seek out a team of physicians specializing in cleft palate care. These teams are often located in cleft palate clinics in larger hospitals. They are sometimes called *craniofacial* teams because they deal with both the head and the face. A team allows for systematic and comprehensive planning in the long-term care of your child. Each member of the team brings his or her special training and experience to bear in the reconstruction of your child's mouth or lip.

After each team member has tested and assessed your child, she brings that information and suggestions for care to the team

15

meeting. Each member gives input, and the team discusses options for care until a plan is formed. The team coordinator, often the lead plastic surgeon, then discusses these options and plans with you. Each team member will work with your child in the area of his specialty. The plastic surgeon will perform surgery, the pediatric dentist may remove teeth that have erupted in the wrong area of the mouth, and the ENT (ear, nose, and throat specialist) will implant any ear tubes necessary for proper ear drainage. Early in your child's care, you may meet with only one or two of the professionals on the team, including the plastic surgeon and ENT. As your child gets older, you may meet with more and more of the team. Often your child will not be seen by the entire cleft palate clinic until close to her second birthday.

Reverend Jesse Jackson, Politician and Activist

A defender of human rights and an African American role model, Jackson has dedicated his life to championing those who are discriminated against. He has acted as a watchdog in American politics for decades. Like Stacy Keach (see page 13), Jackson generally wears a mustache that hides any scarring.

Who Is on the Team?

Because your child's cleft reconstruction may involve not only the closure of lip or palate clefts, but also dental work, speech correction, and psychological help, among other things, there are many professionals who may be included on a cleft palate team. These professionals may work in some of the following fields:

Plastic Surgery: Plastic surgery deals with the reconstruction or alteration of external defects. The plastic surgeon will do the primary work in lip adhesions, palate reconstruction, rhinoplasty (nose reconstruction), and other reconstructions.

Pediatrics: A pediatrician is a doctor who specializes in the treatment of children.

Otolaryngology: This specialist concentrates his or her practice on the ear and larynx.

Orthodontics: An orthodontist specializes in correcting the placement and positioning of teeth.

Oral/Maxillofacial Surgery: Oral (having to do with the mouth) and maxillofacial (the upper jaw and face) surgery may include work on bone structure.

Prosthodontics: A dentist whose specialty involves the use of oral appliances is a prosthodontist.

Speech and Language Pathology: In this field a certified and/or licensed specialist diagnoses and treats speech disorders and communication irregularities.

Audiology: Audiologists are certified and/or licensed specialists who are trained in the science of hearing. The audiologist measures hearing, diagnoses hearing loss, and works on various remedies for hearing loss including hearing devices or therapies.

Psychology: A certified and/or licensed specialist may work with your child in the area of mental and emotional processes.

Social Services: Case workers and others in the social services may steer your family toward programs to help financially and socially in dealing with your child's impairment. They can be helpful advocates in determining school programming for your child.

Radiology: Radiology involves the use of X rays to diagnose and treat impairments and injuries.

Genetics: The geneticist on the team will help you map any possible hereditary links to your child's cleft presentation.

Nursing: You may speak with the nursing staff more often than any other specialists on the team. The nurses are equipped to answer your questions and act as liaisons between you and the other specialists. These hard-working individuals will care for your child both before and after surgeries, and will be your support system during times of stress.

Your Role on the Team

You have a vital role on the team caring for your child. You have already taken a great step forward in that you are actively seeking information on your child's condition and possible options for care. Never forget, *you are your child's best advocate!* Finding a team of doctors whom you trust is a vital first step. Research the clinic, ask questions of the team coordinator, read information about clefting. Find out the number of cleft reconstructions that the clinic, and the plastic surgeon in particular, have performed. Ask to see photographs of other children on whom they have worked.

If you feel put off by the team coordinator, or uncomfortable with her, it may be advisable to seek out another clinic. Any team leader should take the time to answer your questions thoroughly in language you can understand. If she doesn't, rephrase your question and do not be afraid to tell the doctor you did not understand her answer. Ask her to explain it again. Often a doctor who seems brusque may think that you understand the complex language often used in the medical profession. Once you've made clear your limitations in understanding this language, doctors are often wonderfully patient.

All of the doctors on the team want the very best for your child. It is critical to remember this fact. They sincerely want to work with you to find the best options for your child—and to plan a normal, healthy future for him. Knowing that all of you are working toward that goal is the glue that binds the entire team together.

Once you have found the team, your most important responsibility is communication. Continue to ask questions about your child's care, as well as medical procedures, advances in technology, therapies, and other subjects affecting your child. Report any problems you have observed at home. For example, if you notice food leaking from your child's nose, let the plastic surgeon know. There may be a *fistula* (a small hole) in the hard palate. Do not hesitate to mention anything that concerns you, no matter how insignificant it may seem. This will allow the doctors to address any problems immediately and follow their progress. If there is no problem, you will receive reassurance that your fears are unwarranted.

No doctor is going to laugh at your concern for your child or your confusion about the complexities of treatment. After all, your doctors have had years and years of schooling, hands-on training, and practical experience. You, on the other hand, have just recently been thrust into this world of cleft palate reconstruction, probably with little background or none whatsoever! Continue to ask questions about treatments. Ask the team how you can best aid them in therapy or in pre- and post-surgical care.

The best results for your child will come from your diligence in working with the team. Work with your child's speech therapist; learn the exercises critical to improving your child's speech. Follow post-surgical directions to the letter. If the ENT tells you to put five drops in your child's ear twice a day, do exactly that. Don't change orders for your convenience or skip medications. Another critical aspect of your participation is attending all clinic appointments. The team must see the changes occurring in your child's mouth as your child ages and grows. Skipping appointments only hinders the team in their work. Of course, there may be times of emergency when an appointment must be rescheduled. Do your best to make this an extremely rare occurrence.

You are a valuable and equal member of the team caring for your child. Never feel intimidated by the education and experience of the physicians. Instead, try to see their experience and education as valuable tools for the entire team to use. You bring valuable tools to the team that none of the others can bring: you know your child, her habits, and her temperament better than they ever could. You can see anything out of the ordinary long before any other team member. This information is a critical factor in the team's planning. Continue to work with the team throughout the years of follow-up care. Educate yourself on possible options and advances in care for cleft-affected children. Listen to and talk with the team. Together, you will find the best options for your child's unique plan for a healthy, happy life.

Preliminary Decisions for Surgery

Just as every cleft presentation is different, so, too, are the methods the surgical team will use to repair the defect. The complexity of the surgery is in direct correlation to the severity of the cleft. In the case of a mild presentation, that is, a slight notch-shaped cleft in the lip or a small mark in the palate, surgery may be delayed until the child is older, allowing the child to make the decision to have reconstructive surgery. Some teens and adults may decide to forgo surgery completely, allowing a slight defect to remain.

When the presentation is mild, insurance companies may deny coverage for the repair, considering the surgery cosmetic rather than reconstructive. If your child has a minor cleft that does not affect function in any way, you may want to seek approval from your insurance company before proceeding with surgery. Even a minor presentation will cost thousands of dollars to repair if surgery is warranted.

If the cleft is more severe—if it is disfiguring or it impacts the normal functioning of the mouth—surgery is indeed a viable option for you. Again, the type of surgery depends upon the presentation itself. Some surgeries include lip adhesion, soft palate reconstruction, hard palate reconstruction, bone grafting in the *alveolar ridge* (the part of the jaw that contains the teeth), or rhinoplasty. Additional potential surgeries include *pharyngoplasty*, in which a flap of skin is used to connect the soft palate to the back of the throat; the reparation of fistulas, or small holes, in the hard palate; lip and palate revision; and the installation of ear tubes. At times, presurgical devices may be used to help position parts of the mouth, alveolar ridge, or lip in order to facilitate successful surgery.

The descriptions in this chapter are general. Each surgeon may perform a surgery in a slightly different manner, according to her training and experience. When you have found a cleft palate team, it is your duty to question the surgeon on her methods and the potential results. Find out about the surgeon's experience, credentials, and skills. Most doctors will be happy to show you photographs of children on whom they have operated. Are the results aesthetically pleasing? Is there minimal scarring? The more you know, the better an advocate you can be for your child.

Lip Adhesion

Lip adhesion is simply the closing and suturing of a cleft in the lip. Generally, this surgery will be the first one performed on your child. The team will wait until your baby is past the *neonatal* stage (newborn stage, generally the first month after birth). At approximately 2 to 3 months of age, your child's health and weight will be assessed to see whether he is ready for this surgery. Some children may be too small or too frail to endure the risks of surgery and will have to wait until they are older. The goal of most teams is to have the surgery completed before the child learns to talk, so that normal speech function is facilitated. Additional goals include minimal scarring, a pleasant appearance with a "normal" shape to the lip line, and the potential for normal development of the face. It is hoped that, after lip adhesion surgery, the child will have enough elasticity in the lip to drink, eat, and speak in a normal manner.

The surgery itself may be done in one procedure, although a revision may occur when the child is older to facilitate functionality and a pleasant appearance. Depending on your child's presentation, this surgery may be performed in conjunction with other procedures, such as the implantation of ear tubes, soft palate reconstruction, or rhinoplasty. During the surgery, the skin around the cleft is opened to allow the surgeon to suture the two sides of the cleft together. In the case of a complete cleft, the suture line may curve around the edge of the child's nostril and then extend downward to the lip. A child with a bilateral cleft may have suture lines in the shape of a Y or ones that appear like two lines running downward from each nostril to the lip.

As your child heals, the resultant scars will fade. Some children grow up with no real visible scarring. Others may have a light white line where the cleft was closed. If the scarring is considered disfiguring or too apparent, cosmetic plastic surgery or a revision may be performed when the child is older. This may also be done when the lip does not grow proportionally with the rest of the face.

Soft Palate Reconstruction

Again, the complexity of reconstruction is in direct correlation to the severity of the cleft presentation. Generally speaking, a cleft in the soft palate will almost always need repair. The goal of this surgery is functional: the soft palate is used in eating, speech, and breathing. The soft palate is also used to control the *eustachian tubes*, the air ducts from the middle ear to the back of the throat that allow for ear drainage. An incomplete soft palate may result in speech that lacks normal vocal resonance, problems with *explosive* sounds (sounds produced by air expelled with force, such as *t* or *d*, *p* or *b*), *sleep apnea* (brief cessations of breathing during sleep), difficulty eating, *nasal regurgitation* (expulsion of food or liquids through the nose), chronic ear infections, and other complications.

Soft palate reconstruction may occur any time after the child has passed the neonatal stage and is healthy enough to withstand normal surgical methods. The team may, however, opt to delay the surgery until the child is between 6 and 12 months old, or older. If the surgery is to be performed later, do ask the team about the impact the delay may have on normal speech function. If your child is healthy and strong, it is good to have the palate reconstructed before she begins to speak, so that the entire process will not have to be relearned. Ask the team to explain the reasons behind their decision. Trust that a careful and committed team will strive to make the best decisions possible for the welfare of your child.

Soft palate reconstruction may be performed in conjunction with other procedures including lip adhesion, the implantation of ear tubes, and other reconstructive surgery. The process of repairing the soft palate may include opening already existing tissue, pulling it to the center of the cleft, and suturing it shut. At times, there may be insufficient tissue present. If this is the case, the surgeon may close as much of the cleft as possible in the first surgery, allow it to heal and grow, and then revise the palate at a later date. The presentation of a wide cleft may warrant another procedure to overcome *velopharyngeal* inadequacy—that is, an incomplete closure of the soft palate with the back of the throat.

Hard Palate Reconstruction

The goal of hard palate reconstruction is to improve the function of the mouth in eating and speaking. The surgery, in conjunction with speech therapy, is your child's best hope for intelligible speech. The hard palate may be repaired any time after the baby is past the neonatal stage of development. Often this surgery is delayed until after 6 months and even until 12 or 18 months of age. It may be done in conjunction with surgery on the soft palate or other revisions, and is often performed in two or more steps. Methods vary for closing the hard palate. Often, the skin of the gum line or edges of existing hard palate tissue is pulled across the existing cleft and sutured together. This may result in the slight movement of some tooth buds, a situation easily rectified once the baby teeth begin to emerge.

At times, depending on the width of the cleft, complete closure is not possible for a number of years. Fistulas may develop and require additional surgery; this is discussed later in the chapter. Some physicians may use a prosthetic device to cover the cleft before and between surgeries. This device is called an *obtu-rator* and may or may not be used by your team. It can aid in your child's ability to eat and speak until the hard palate has been reconstructed.

Submucous Clefts

A submucous cleft is generally not apparent at birth because it is usually covered by a layer of skin. The team will monitor the child with a submucous cleft and evaluate his progress in general functionality, eating, speaking, and hearing. Surgery to repair a submucous cleft is deemed necessary when there is any evidence of problems in the development and function of the mouth. This surgery can occur at any time after the neonatal stage of development. Submucous cleft repair may consist of opening the tissue of the soft or hard palate, closing the cleft in the muscles above the tissue, then suturing the cleft shut.

Bone Grafts and Alveolar Ridge Reconstruction

As with any procedure, there are several methods of surgery proven to be effective in reconstructing the *alveolar ridge*—the bony ridge on the upper (and lower) portion of the jaw, containing the teeth. Bone may be harvested from any number of areas on your child's body, including the skull or the hip, to be inserted into the cleft area. In some cases, bone marrow is used in the procedure. The complexity of this procedure may necessitate the use of presurgical devices, orthodontics, or other dental work. Generally speaking, the timing of a bone graft operation is determined by the maturity of the child's dental growth. Ideally, the procedure will occur before the eruption of permanent teeth in the cleft-affected area, although there may be great success even after full eruption of these teeth. The team orthodontist, dentist, and surgeons will collaborate on the planning and preparation for this phase of reconstruction.

After the operation, your child may be required to use protective devices to ensure healing. These may include crutches, braces, or helmets. In general, your child will be encouraged to avoid games or activities that require heavy physical exertion or the risk of having her surgical areas bumped. The time frame for healing will depend on the severity of the cleft, the type of procedure used to reconstruct the alveolar ridge, and the health of your child.

The Nose

Children born with a cleft of the lip will often have a distended or deformed nose. Depending on the presentation of the cleft, nasal surgery may be performed at the same time as a lip adhesion. Further reconstruction and revision of the nose may be performed in the subsequent stages of cleft reconstruction. Many teams proceed with rhinoplasty only after the child's nasal growth is complete. Some teams take into consideration the effect that teasing may have on a child once he enters school, advocating additional surgery in order to facilitate a more normal appearance. If the nasal airway is compromised by a flattened or distended nose, additional surgery may be warranted earlier. This may be accomplished with a much less intrusive surgery than the palate repair. It may even be done on an outpatient basis with few external incisions.

The Ears

If your child has a cleft presentation that affects only her lip, more than likely the ears will not be affected in any way. However, if there is a clefting of the soft palate, the muscles controlling the eustachian tubes may be affected. These tubes connect the middle ear to the pharynx (the part of the alimentary canal between the mouth and esophagus), allowing for drainage and the equalization of pressure on both sides of the eardrum. Each time a person swallows or yawns, the muscles of the soft palate control the pressure on the eardrum through the eustachian tubes. Improper muscle function or the lack of muscle function in the soft palate directly affects the ability of the ear to drain and to equalize pressure. As a result, bacteria causing ear infections may settle into the middle ear.

Some cleft-affected children experience chronic ear infections, resulting in a temporary disruption in hearing. Most children who have chronic ear infections during the first months of life hear the world as though they are under water—sound is literally reaching them through the collected liquid in the middle ear. Most of these children will experience no permanent hearing loss if the problem is rectified early. Some children may have slight to moderate hearing loss as a result of a soft palate cleft.

The ENT on your team will advise you as to the best remedy for improper functioning of the eustachian tubes. More than likely, tubes will be placed in the eardrums during one of the early reconstructive surgeries. This will allow for proper drainage of the fluids in the middle ear. There are different types of tubes, including a standard tube, which is small and straight with a ridge on each end to aid in retaining its placement in the eardrum, used for children who experience chronic ear infections with or without clefts. This tube is less permanent than some other types of tubes and may fall out after time or can easily be removed. Another, more permanent, type of tube has a T-shaped design. In some rare cases, children experience relief of pressure with a simple notch cut into the eardrum.

You will be advised of the proper care for your child's tubes once they are in place. This will often include the use of earplugs during bathing and swimming. Drops are used in the ear for a time after surgery to ensure the tubes do not become blocked. If the tubes do become blocked, it is usually possible to remedy the situation with eardrops. It is seldom necessary to perform additional invasive procedures or replace the tubes. Continued follow-up care at each team screening will help to head off any problems with the tubes. The ENT will check for blockage and correct placement of the tubes, and the speech and language professionals will use various tests to screen for any hearing loss. If hearing loss does occur, it may be overcome with the use of hearing aids and other devices.

Additional Surgeries

As previously mentioned, a wide cleft presentation in the soft palate may result in velopharyngeal inadequacy, a lack of closure between the soft palate and the back of the throat. This may cause serious speech problems—particularly with certain explosive sounds—that cannot be overcome by speech therapy alone. Velopharyngeal inadequacy may be diagnosed using a variety of tests, ranging from simple speech therapy to the use of a small camera inserted via a tube through your child's nose. The camera allows speech professionals to watch the function of the soft palate on a monitor. The procedure is relatively painless, but can be annoying to the young child; you may be asked to hold her still on your lap while the tube is in place.

Your child's speech therapist and plastic surgeon will determine if it is necessary to intervene with additional surgery, the most common of which is a *pharyngoplasty*. This type of repair consists of the construction of a small bridge of tissue connecting the soft palate to the back of the throat, called a *pharyngeal flap*. Some surgeons use a modification of this procedure by bringing in tissue from the sides of the throat. The ultimate result is similar to that of the standard flap procedure: the opening to the throat is made smaller, allowing for proper closure for sound production.

Repairing a Fistula

In many cleft presentations, complete repair of the hard palate is possible in one surgery. For some, additional surgery may be necessary to close small holes called *fistulas*. These holes may be allowed to remain until the repair of the alveolar ridge. Some may be so insignificant as to never require surgery. However, if there is nasal leakage of food or if the fistula affects speech, surgery may be warranted. Closing a fistula is similar to the original hard palate reconstruction, but the surgery is of a much smaller scale.

Later Surgeries

Other surgeries may include revisions of the original surgery to lessen scarring and aid in proper functioning. These procedures may be performed at any time during your child's development—or even during the adult years. Many adults have had lip revisions performed in order to give themselves a more natural appearance. However, the improvements in plastic surgery over the years have made many lip revisions unnecessary, with scars often nearly invisible. Adult lip revision may be considered cosmetic surgery by some insurance companies and may not be covered. This should be investigated and promises of coverage should be put in writing before the procedure is undergone. The professionals on your team will advise you of any recommendations for further surgical procedures.

Cheech Marin, Actor, Comedian, and Writer

Born Richard Marin in 1946, Cheech Marin has made a name as a comedian (as part of Cheech and Chong), writer (eight films, including Up in Smoke *and* Born in East LA*), and actor (*Spy Kids, Luminarias, Tin Cup, *"Nash Bridges,"* Up in Smoke, *and more). He has made guest appearances on "South Park," "Sex and the City," "Tracey Takes On..." and many other television programs. Marin has appeared on screen with a mustache and without, his scar seeming to have no affect on his entertainment appeal.*

Preparing Your Child for Surgery

As you begin the process of reconstruction and revision, be sure that you understand clearly each procedure. Do not be afraid to ask your doctors to explain each step of the surgery to you, from the presurgical physical and testing, to the procedure itself, to follow-up care and check-ups. You must also completely understand your role in each of these phases of care. You will then be equipped to give your child the best care at home and in the hospital, and, in the case of an older child, be able to answer his questions and prepare him for surgery and recovery.

Talking to Your Child about Surgery

As your child gets older and is able to understand the fact that she has a cleft lip or palate, you will be able to explain more about the procedures involved in reconstructing the cleft. Give information only as necessary to the very young child and in terms she will understand. Try not to frighten or confuse your child with big, medical—and scary-sounding—terms. You may want to tell your child that when she was born she had a "broken" part on her mouth. Tell her that the doctors are going to fix it in the hospital.

Don't burden your child with lists of future surgeries or what they may entail. Focus on the current issues. However, if your child asks about future procedures, you should be honest. You may tell him that you would like to focus on this surgery but that there may be others in the future. It is critical that you answer every question with honesty. Don't try to make your child less afraid by telling him "it won't hurt a bit." This may be true of the surgery itself, but he *will* be uncomfortable in recovery. Your child may then be less likely to trust you in the future.

Explain each step in the surgical procedure. For example:

* First you will get a check-up. The doctors and nurses will weigh you and measure you. Then they will take a blood test. They will use a small needle, like a shot, and take a very small amount of blood. They want to be sure you are very healthy before the surgery. The doctor will talk to you and me about the surgery. You may ask questions when the doctor talks to us. Next we will go to the hospital early in the morning (or name the time). You will not be able to eat or drink anything before the surgery. That is to keep you safe during surgery in case you feel a little sick. At the hospital, a nurse may weigh you again. The nurse will listen to your

heart and take your blood pressure. You will change into some hospital pajamas. I will be with you all of this time.

* The nurse might give you some medicine to drink. The medicine might make you feel a little sleepy or goofy. It will help your body to get ready for the surgery. I will wait with you until it is time for you to go into the operating room. (Some hospitals allow parents to enter the operating theater with their child. If this is the case, include this information. *Do not* promise to be there with your child as they are put to sleep if you are not sure you will be able to. Broken promises breed mistrust.) A person called an anesthesiologist will then help you to fall asleep. He or she will put a special plastic mask over your face. In just a couple of seconds you will fall asleep. (Again, be sure to question your team about the exact methods used so that you can be truthful with your child.)

* When you wake up, the operation will be all finished. You might wake up with a nurse. If I am not there, the nurse will come and get me once you are awake. I will be waiting in a special room until you are awake. There will be some special machines around your bed. There might be a blood pressure cuff on your arm. There might be a plastic tube taped to your hand that leads to a plastic bag full of what looks like water. That is a special type of medicine. You might have the plastic tube on your hand for a couple of days. You will hear beeping and other sounds around you. The beeping will be your heartbeat on a machine. Other machines might be beeping with the sounds of other people's heartbeats. None of these sounds is scary. The machines help the nurses and doctors make sure everyone is safe and healthy.

* You might then be moved to a special room where nurses can watch you carefully. I will be with you. Once you are ready, you can be moved into a regular hospital room. You might have a roommate or you might be the only child in the room.

No matter what, I can be with you. I will sleep in the room with you, too! I can sleep on a special chair that opens into a little bed.

* Your mouth might feel sore or uncomfortable for a few days. The nurses will bring you special medicine to help you with the uncomfortable feeling.

* The nurses will check on you often. They will check your heart and your mouth. They might take your blood pressure. They might give you medicine on some of their visits. They will even bring your meals right to your room!

* When the surgery is over, you will have finished one more step in having your mouth fixed! We can look in a mirror and see what the doctor did on the outside or the roof of your mouth. Your brothers and sisters can visit you once you are feeling strong enough. (Mention any other relatives or friends who are planning to visit.) After a day or two in the hospital, we will go home!

Add as much detail to your story as you think your child may need. Keep your conversation positive and cheerful. Continually focus on how much the surgery will help your child's appearance or speech. Assure him that it is normal to be nervous but that the doctors and nurses have taken care of hundreds of children like him and they will do their very best to take good care of him. Repeatedly assure your child of your presence. You may tell him that you won't be in the operating room but you will be in a room nearby. Your assurances and confidence will have a direct effect on how well your child handles his own fears.

Decisions

Whenever possible, allow your child some control of her situation by giving her the opportunity to make decisions. With a small child, the decisions may be over simple things such as which books or videos to pack, or whether to wear the hospital pajamas or her own (be sure to check hospital policy on this). An older child may be able to have some input regarding the surgery itself. Should she have a lip revision done on a scar, or, after you discuss the procedure and possible results, would she like to wait—or not have the procedure at all? Allow your child the opportunity to question, understand, and decide on anything that is age appropriate. Some control over her situation will go far in easing her fears and feelings of powerlessness. Be aware that some children will balk out of fear at having a procedure. If a surgery is deemed necessary by you and the team, explain to your child that you understand his reluctance, but that the procedure must be done for his benefit. Carefully explain the procedure and the desired results. Focus attention on how his quality of life will improve once the surgery has been performed. Do not give your child veto power over necessary surgeries. This is not healthy and may cause many difficulties for him in the future.

Rewards or Bribes

There is nothing wrong with promising your child some special gift or surprise to be given after the surgery. This can be a positive thing for your child to focus on when feeling afraid. One parent gave her son a new hand-held video game to play in the hospital room. The boy looked forward to having the coveted game so much that he was eager to have the surgery, asking daily for the time remaining until "hospital day." Explain to your child that the new book, game, or toy you will be giving her is to help her pass the time in the hospital after surgery. Rewards may cross the line into unhealthy bribes if you find that you cannot get your child to cooperate with doctors without a gift or treat. Avoid falling into this expensive trap. Explain to your child that cooperating with the doctors will help them to do their very best for her. Let her know that you will not tolerate behavior that interrupts the team's plan for her care. Remember that the best reward you can give your child is a huge hug and kiss, along with the words "I love you, and I am so proud of you!"

Tom Brokaw, Television News Personality

According to the Wide Smiles website's "Wondering Who Is Affected by a Cleft?" Brokaw was born with a cleft. He does, indeed, have an unusual presentation in his upper lip that is reminiscent of a bilateral cleft scar.

Familiarity as an Ally

The more familiar your child is with the hospital and staff, the more comfortable he will feel during his stay. Talk to the hospital staff about a possible tour of the facility. Show your child the type of room in which he will stay. Walk through the hallways, and play in the pediatric playroom if there is one. Eat lunch or have a snack in the cafeteria. Walk the grounds. Some hospitals may even have a formal tour during which your child may visit the operating room and recovery room. Allow your child time to meet a nurse or two (without interrupting the nurses' busy work schedule).

Young children can play-act scenarios at home with a toy doctor bag. Take turns being the patient and the doctor. Pay attention to the things your child says. This is a good way for him to voice his fears without having to "admit" them. If the pretend patient talks obsessively about pain, you can, as the pretend doctor, assure him that the uncomfortable feeling will go away once he drinks "medicine." Then offer your child a small drink of juice. Play-acting helps your child face the situation and allows him to rehearse possible solutions.

Another way to assure and calm your child is to educate her. Go to your local library and check out books on hospitals. Read children's stories on clefting (such as the one in this book). Rent or purchase videos in which your child's favorite characters visit the hospital. Look up sites on the Internet. One of the best websites available is that of Wide Smiles, at widesmiles.org. This site includes information on virtually every aspect of clefting. It even has a photo gallery of children who were born with clefts. Many of the photographs chronicle the children's development through various procedures. Anything that helps your child feel comfortable and unafraid is a valuable tool in keeping her concerns at bay. Be sure to pack that special stuffed toy or blanket. Having it along for the hospital stay will give her extra comfort and a tangible reminder of home.

Lee Raymond, CEO Exxon-Mobil

According to sources at The American Cleft Palate Association, Raymond was born with a cleft presentation. A powerful and astute businessman, Raymond has evidence of a cleft scar on his lip.

Preparing Yourself for Your Child's Surgery

A Hospital Tour in Words

Registration: Most likely, you will preregister your child. The registration forms will ask for billing information, insurance information, your mailing address, and the nature of your child's admittance to the hospital. You may ask the representatives to clarify what information is required and give the reasons it is needed. You may expect to spend as little as 15 minutes or as long as an hour on registration procedures.

Preoperative Procedures: Preoperative testing is necessary to ensure that your child's surgery will be safe and successful. Height, weight, blood pressure, and heart rate will be measured, and blood tests taken. X rays, ultrasound tests, bone density tests, or other tests may be required for some of the more complex surgeries. Generally, you will be present with your child for these tests. On the day of the surgery, several general tests will again be performed including blood pressure and heart rate. Your team may ask for any pediatric records from your child's primary physician. In general, each of the doctors who will be participating in the surgery will speak with you briefly about what his or her part of the procedure will be. This is the perfect time to ask any last-minute questions you may have.

Handing Over Your Child: Once you have gone over the pre-operative procedures, the anesthesiologist will confer with you. She may give your child an oral drug or a shot to begin the procedure. Your child will become sleepy or slightly tipsy. You will be allowed to remain with your child until the anesthesiologist is ready to begin. Many hospitals allow the parent to carry the child into the operating room and remain with him until he is asleep.

Surgical Waiting: The surgical waiting area may be a small, quiet room or it may be a large, lobby-like area in which dozens of families are passing time. You will be escorted to this area. Often there are magazines, televisions, coffee, and other items there for your convenience. You may consider bringing along that novel you meant to finish or a needlework project to pass the time. A staff person is often readily available to answer questions or check on your child's progress. He can also give you information about pastoral care.

Pastoral Care: Many hospitals have counselors, pastors, or priests who are available to speak with you. They can visit your child's room or even sit a while with you in the surgical waiting area. These compassionate individuals are there to help you through this difficult time. It is not an imposition to ask to speak with one of them, and you may find that they are of immense help.

The Surgeon's Visit: After the surgery, the physicians will speak briefly with you about what occurred in the operating and recovery rooms. Sometimes only one surgeon will speak with you, but if there are several working with your child that day, they may all speak with you.

Recovery: After the surgery, your child will go to a recovery room. There may be several patients in the room in various stages of consciousness. You may be taken from the surgical waiting area to the recovery room to be with your child. The length of time your child spends there will depend on her condition, the procedure, and the availability of rooms on the pediatric wing. Remember that this is a quiet place where any sudden noise may startle those awakening from surgery.

Pediatric Intensive Care Unit (PICU): Because your child's procedures are generally performed in the mouth area, she may be placed in the intensive care unit. This allows the medical staff to watch her more closely for swelling or obstructions. It does not, in most cases, mean that your child is in grave danger. If a problem does arise, however, the intensive care staff can intervene immediately. Be aware that the staff will answer your questions and do everything they can to help you and your child during your stay in the PICU. They will not, however, discuss the cases of the other children around you. Generally, you can stay in the PICU with your child as long as your presence is not disruptive. Your stay in the PICU may be as short as a few hours or could be close to 24 hours.

Pediatric Hospital Unit: The pediatric wings of a hospital may be divided into "Big" (older children) and "Little" (younger children). As your child grows stronger, he or she may be moved into a regular pediatric room, where he may have a roommate. You may stay with your child in the pediatric room. For times when you need to leave (to eat, take a shower, etc.), many hospitals have "cuddlers"—volunteers who will remain with your child while you are out of the room. Nurses and doctors will visit your child periodically to keep track of his vital signs and dispense medicine. Do not be afraid to ask questions. Also, it is fine to ask the nurses and doctors to introduce themselves to your child before touching him.

Psychological Preparation

As you prepare your child, you will find comfort for yourself as well. The more you learn about the procedure, the hospital, and the staff, the more you will be able to calm many of your own fears. While every surgery involves certain risk factors, be assured that problems with this kind of surgery are extremely rare and generally easily remedied. It is normal to be nervous about your child's surgery; try to use this concern in positive ways. It may be the catalyst in your own education process, spurring you to learn all you can about clefting and reconstructive surgery. It may help you to become an advocate for your child and other children.

No matter how much you know about the process, you should seek out other people whom you trust and can talk to. Communicating your concerns, venting your frustrations, and releasing your grief are vital to your personal health. Keep the lines of communication open with your spouse or significant other. Listen to his or her concerns without being judgmental or trying to offer solutions—unless you are asked to do so. Ask him or her to show you this same courtesy. If your companion is not comfortable hearing your concerns, you may wish to seek out another person in whom you can confide. A trusted friend or a counselor is a good choice.

Acknowledge the fact that each person is unique, and that each person will handle grief and fear in a different manner. Some need to talk about every detail. Others remain silent and reflective. Some cry; others may not. There is no right or wrong way to grieve the losses inflicted by having a child with an impairment. There is no time limit on this type of pain, either. You and your spouse or significant other may rebound into a new stage of grief with each subsequent surgery. This is normal. However, if your fears or grief turn into depression, or hinder normal functioning for a length of time, it is best to seek out professional help. These issues are discussed further in subsequent chapters.

Post-Operative Care for Your Child

Before leaving the hospital after a surgery, be sure you understand all aspects of your child's home care. How is medicine to be dispensed? What therapies are involved? When should your child be seen again for a post-operative check-up? The nurse who discharges your child will go over these requirements carefully. Ask questions about anything you feel unsure about. The most important factors in your child's successful recovery at home are your love and support and your ability to follow postoperative directions. In rare instances, complications may arise at home. If your child runs a fever, complains of pain that cannot be relieved, or begins to bleed, contact your physician immediately.

Once you are home, set up a bed for your child in a quiet area where you can be readily available to her. Remember, she will need more sleep than normal while recovering from surgery. Roughhousing with other siblings may cause pain and, even worse, damage to the newly reconstructed areas. A television and VCR or DVD player, as well as books, art supplies, toys, and games, can help your child pass the time. Keep visitors to a minimum during the first few days, until your child has had time to adjust. Exhausting her with a constant barrage of people will only hinder her recovery.

You may need to ask for a few days off from your job in order to adequately care for your child. Before the surgery, check with your human resources department about a leave of absence. Know your employer's policies concerning leaves and arrange one to start the day your child returns home. Use the help offered by friends and family members. Accept meals. Allow someone to clean your house for you. Focus your time and attention on your child. You may also wish to find a friend or relative who can give some of their time in caring for your child. If you have no extended family or friends and feel overwhelmed, contact a church or mission group, mental health organization, support group, or referral service. Explain the situation and ask for help. You may be surprised at others' compassion and willingness to help you.

CHAPTER 3

Feeding the Cleft-Affected Child

Breast Milk or Formula?

Consult your doctor in order to make the best decision for your child. It has long been acknowledged that breast milk is the perfect food for an infant. It provides both nourishment and protection from illness in the early days of life. Some studies have shown that the use of breast milk may be instrumental in reducing the frequency and severity of ear infections, to which children with clefts in the soft palate are prone. Modern formula has been enhanced and can be virtually as healthful as breast milk. The choices of formula range from soy-based to iron-enriched products. Your baby's doctor will be able to help you choose the formula suited to your baby's needs. Many mothers choose a combination of breast milk and formula. This allows the nursing mother some rest time, but may cause some babies to lose interest in the breast.

If, because of the cleft presentation, your child cannot nurse, you may still be able to obtain breast milk for your child by hand-expressing or pumping. Many insurance companies even cover the cost of breast pumps in the case of a child with a cleft palate. (You may need a prescription from your doctor or a letter from the cleft palate team stating their recommendation for your child's use of breast milk.) Special bottles and nipples for the baby who cannot nurse will be discussed later in this chapter. In some cases, children with cleft palates may be able to nurse adequately with the use of a prosthetic device. This device fits over the cleft in the palate, sealing the area in order to facilitate sucking. Parents may discuss this option with the cleft palate team.

Breast-feeding the Newborn

Feeding a baby with a cleft may be frightening to the new parent, even one who has had other children. Along with those fears may be doubts about your ability to succeed, or, perhaps, sadness at being unable to nurse your baby. Such doubts may be unwarranted, however, depending on the presentation of your child's cleft. You may be able to successfully nurse your child if the cleft is only in the lip or gum, or is too small to affect the sucking function of the soft palate. In the case of a lip or gum cleft, you may be able to place your finger over the cleft, allowing your baby to latch onto the nipple and suck. If the soft palate has just a small cleft, your baby may have little difficulty in nursing. A nurse or a lactation consultant may be able to explore with you the possibility of nursing your baby, helping you experiment with various positions and styles.

Your desire or ability to nurse, the choice between using formula and pumping breast milk, and the frequency of feeding are all decisions that are unique to your family's needs and the needs of your baby. These decisions should not be based solely on whether or not your child has a cleft palate. The feeding needs of a child with a cleft are the same as those of a child without a cleft. The only difference may be that one child can suck while another may not be able to, or that a baby with a cleft will have to be positioned differently to prevent milk from moving incorrectly.

Support for the Breast-feeding or Expressing Mother

It is vital that you have the support of those around you as you learn to nurse or express breast milk for your baby. The hospital or your doctor's office may be able to recommend a lactation consultant to coach you through breast-feeding or expressing your milk. Her role is to help you have the most successful feeding experience possible for both you and your baby. She will be able to answer any questions you may have and give you information about breast milk and its benefits. Many lactation consultants, however, may not have experience with helping to nurse a child with a cleft palate. A good consultant will admit her lack of knowledge but search out options and answers for you. It is important that you feel comfortable with your lactation consultant in order to cultivate a calm, relaxed environment for nursing your baby.

The support of your spouse or significant other, as well as those extended family members whose opinions you value, may also have an impact on whether or not you feel calm and capable. Comments such as "You can't nurse that baby" or "Why are you working so hard on this? Wouldn't it be easier to just feed him with a bottle?" can be damaging. You may be able to change the attitudes of those around you by asking for their help. Make requests that address your needs and emotions without attacking the other party. For example, you may begin with: "I am really struggling with nursing my baby. This is important to me because it is so healthy for the baby. I would really appreciate your help in this. I need encouragement and a positive environment in order to be successful. Because I value your opinions so much, you can be my best source of support." Your lactation consultant, physician, and even counselor or minister may be able to help you enlist the support of those around you.

Remember that nursing takes practice and time. Your baby has never done this before. Allow both yourself and your baby time to "get it right." Many babies who have no physical defects have difficulty nursing in the beginning; your child may need a bit more practice before she finds the correct technique. Your ability to remain patient and calm will help your baby to remain calm. If you find you and your baby are having trouble, or don't seem to be "catching on," ask the lactation consultant or your doctor for other options.

Preparing to Nurse

Some women prepare their breasts for nursing even before the baby is born. Rubbing your nipples with a terry cloth towel may help to prepare them for the sucking pressure from your baby or a breast pump. Lotions and oils to keep the nipples tender may also be used, especially if your nipples become raw or sore from nursing or pumping. Be sure that the lotions you use are safe for the baby, and that your nipples are clean and dry before nursing or pumping. Any discomfort you may have will generally be short-lived, however; most women become accustomed to nursing or pumping within a short amount of time.

When preparing to nurse or express milk, cultivate a calm environment. Try dimming the lights and playing soft music. Tension may make the situation more difficult, causing you to become even more tense. Try to maintain an attitude of learning and practice. Applaud yourself for any step forward in this area…even if the step was simply to try. You may want to massage your breasts or apply hot packs or warm cloths for about 15 to 20 minutes before nursing. A warm shower or bath before nursing will have a dual benefit: it will help relax you, and the warmth can help with the "letdown reflex" which causes your milk to begin flowing. (Many women feel a tingle or slight release with the letdown reflex; others report feeling nothing significant.) You may even hand-express some milk to help begin the flow or use a manual or electric breast pump.

You will want to feed or express frequently in the first few weeks in order to build an adequate milk supply. Experts recommend nursing or pumping every 2 to 3 hours. As you work to establish your milk supply, remember to increase your own intake of fluid. Each time your baby drinks, have a tall glass of water. Keep a pitcher readily available, or invest in a supply of bottled water.

Joaquin Phoenix, Actor

Rising star and brother of the late River Phoenix, Joaquin Phoenix has made a name for himself in movies such as To Die For, Quills, and Gladiator. Often portraying villains, Phoenix has a mark characteristic of a unilateral cleft scar.

Nursing Positions

The position you choose should provide ample support for your baby. You may use pillows and other soft items to help you support your child; a footstool is also helpful. Be aware that nursing a baby takes some time—20 to 30 minutes or more once a child learns to nurse—so both of you need to be comfortable. The traditional position of cradling your baby in one arm may not be the best for a child with a soft palate cleft, in that milk can leak into the baby's nose, possibly causing him to choke. However, this position is fine for children with lip or gum clefts. It allows you to easily place a finger over the cleft, sealing the gap and allowing your child to latch onto the breast.

A more upright position is recommended for babies with palate clefts. In a modified "football" hold, your baby is held facing you. One hand holds the baby's head (and may be supported by pillows) while the other guides the nipple into the baby's mouth. Your baby will be positioned similarly to a football in the hands of a running back. In a variation on this position, your baby faces you and straddles your abdomen. The use of pillows and a footstool enable you to keep the baby upright without stress on your arms.

Even in an upright position, your baby may have some nasal regurgitation. This will not harm your baby, although he may sneeze or choke until he becomes more accustomed to it. As your baby grows older he will be able to move food more efficiently to the back of his mouth, diminishing the likelihood of nasal regurgitation.

Bottle-feeding the Newborn

After consulting your doctor, you may decide that bottle-feeding is the viable option for your situation. Research the various types of formula available to you. Do not be alarmed if you have to try a number of different brands before finding the one that best suits your infant. Your baby's doctor will help you with this process. He will also help you find the correct type of bottle and nipple to use with your child's cleft presentation. These options will be discussed in greater detail later in this chapter.

Once you make an informed decision to use formula, do not let the opinions of others pressure you to change your mind or make you feel guilty. This decision is personal and must be made with consideration of your individual situation. Relatives or friends who pressure you about your decision may be told that you carefully considered every option, discussing it with your baby's doctors, and decided that bottle-feeding or formula is the best possible option for you and your baby. To diffuse hurt feelings you may even thank the person for their concern, telling them you appreciate that they are concerned about the well-being of your baby, just as you are.

When Your Baby Cannot Nurse: The Emotional Issues

The emotional impact of being unable to nurse your child can be strong. You may feel a mixture of emotions such as guilt, anger, and sadness. These are typical emotions associated with the grieving process, through which you must travel. Be aware that this is a normal process and that every person grieves in a unique manner. You may find it helpful to talk about your feelings with your spouse or significant other, a trusted friend, a pastor, or a counselor. Keep in mind these most important facts: this is not your fault and you can still have a perfect bond with your baby. The bonding experience is built through time spent nurturing your child, regardless of whether the breast or the bottle is used. As you cuddle and feed your baby, she learns trust and love. She learns that your gentle touch and your voice belong to someone who loves her and will take care of her. You, in turn, will fall more and more in love with the delightful little creature you are holding.

Bottle-feeding Positions

The positioning of your baby for bottle-feeding is similar to that for nursing: a more upright position will help reduce nasal regurgitation. The cradle position may be modified by using pillows to raise the baby's back and head. Some babies learn to bottle feed in a near sitting position. You can use one hand to stabilize your baby's head and chin while the other holds the bottle. Pillows can support the baby's back. The modified "football" hold and straddle position both work well with a bottle.

Some mothers have great success in leaning the baby's back against their chest in a semi-reclining position. It is important to observe the baby, however, to catch any choking or other problems. It is NEVER recommended that you prop a bottle for your child. This is dangerous in that your attention may waver and your child may choke on a constant flow of milk. Whatever positions you choose should be based on both your and your baby's comfort and ability to feed efficiently. You may find that your baby prefers one position to another.

Expressing Breast Milk

Using a breast pump or hand expressing your milk may be necessary when your child's cleft presentation does not allow for adequate sucking. This is often the case with babies with a bilateral cleft. You may also wish to use a pump to supplement nursing, allowing you to have a ready supply of breast milk for a bottle-feeding. Hand expressing milk may seem more natural and certainly can be accomplished. It does, however, have a tendency to be much more time consuming and not as efficient as the pumps.

If you choose to hand express, be sure that you wash your hands thoroughly with a disinfectant soap. Wash and dry the breast. Use a collection reservoir that is large enough to collect any misguided spray of milk. A bowl or larger cup will suffice. Follow the steps explained above in "Preparing to Nurse." Once you have established the letdown reflex, gently apply pressure to the areola (the dark circle around the nipple) and nipple area of the breast, pulling gently outward. At first you may notice only a bead of milk that drips down the breast or onto your fingers. Continue practicing until you can establish fine sprays. Empty one breast and then turn your attention to the other.

Manual pumps, which may be provided by your hospital, are a bit more efficient in harvesting your milk supply. These pumps have a reservoir, tubing, a "nipple shell," and a pump handle. The nipple shell is placed over the breast. You then move the pump handle in and out until adequate suction has been established. Within moments you will notice milk draining through the tubes into the reservoir. You should finish one breast and then move on to the other. While this is an efficient means to express breast milk, it can take quite a bit of time, and the manual pumping action may tire your arm.

Electric pumps are far more efficient. They come in smaller portable models that can be purchased and in larger models that may be rented from hospitals and medical supply companies. If your hospital does have a supply of electric breast pumps, often you will need a written prescription from your doctor to rent one. Insurance companies often cover the rental completely or in part when you provide them with a copy of the prescription and/or a letter from the physician explaining your baby's situation. If it's available, opt for the dual breast pump. This machine allows for expressing milk from both breasts at the same time. It significantly reduces the amount of time you must spend pumping milk.

Breast milk should be stored in glass containers, as there is some evidence that the chemicals in plastic containers leech into the milk. The milk can be frozen and may be thawed in the refrigerator overnight. Once thawed, the milk should be warmed under a flow of warm water or in a standing pan or bowl of warm water from the tap. *Do not* microwave the milk or heat it on the stove. Serious injury may result.

Equipment for Bottle-Feeding

A number of types of nipples and bottles are readily available, from those of standard manufacture to those designed with a cleft-affected child in mind. Standard nipples such as NUK nipples may be used by babies with a cleft without any alteration at all. At times an X-shaped crosscut may be added to the nipple to allow for adequate flow. Older parents of adults who were born with clefts may insist you purchase a lamb's nipple, available at farm supply stores. While this nipple does allow for easier feeding of a cleft-affected child, there are many other options available. When choosing a nipple, take into account its length. It must make contact with the palate and tongue but not be so long as to cause your baby to gag.

Three of the most common cleft palate feeders are the Mead Johnson C.P. Nurser, the Ross C.P. Nurser, and the Haberman Feeder. These can be purchased from a medical supply store or directly from the manufacturers.

* The Mead Johnson C.P. Nurser consists of an elongated, rounded nipple on a soft-bodied bottle. The nipple allows for correct contact with the palate and tongue and the soft bottle enables the parent to squeeze the formula at varied rates.

* The Ross C.P. Nurser consists of a hard-bodied bottle and a special nipple. The nipple consists of a tube that tapers at the end. It allows for a steady dripping of milk. Sucking pressure from the baby can increase the flow.

* The Haberman Feeder has a hard plastic bottle that resem-

bles a large test tube. It has graduated measurement lines and a special reservoir in the nipple. The nipple looks like a continuation of the bottle except it is soft and is tapered at the end. The reservoir and valve system allows smaller amounts of milk or formula to enter the long nipple. The baby may chew down on the end of the nipple or apply sucking pressure to regulate the flow; the parent can also apply pressure to regulate the flow.

Your child may need to begin feeding with a special cleft palate feeder but be able to move on to a standard bottle and nipple as he grows older and stronger. Squeezable bottles and platex nursers that include a plastic bag allow you to control the flow of milk by applying pressure, and may be a good choice among the varieties of standard bottles. Your physician or craniofacial team can help you to decide which method of bottle-feeding works best for your child.

Transferring from Bottle to Breast

If an initial surgery closes or partially closes a palate cleft, and you have maintained a milk supply, it is possible to switch your child from bottle-feeding to breast-feeding. This will take the same type of patience and relaxed atmosphere you cultivated when first teaching your child to eat. Some babies fuss over the sudden change. They may find that eating from a bottle was easier than breast-feeding, that it required less physical effort on their part. However, with patience and practice, breast-feeding can become a viable option. Once again, you may use the help of a lactation consultant or specialist in learning to nurse your baby. Don't put too much pressure on yourself or your child to find immediate success. As with any learned skill, this may take time and effort.

Frequency of Feeding

There are many different theories on how frequently an infant should be fed. Some factions insist that feeding on demand is the only way to have a happy and healthy baby. Others insist that infants should begin to follow a schedule when very young. Your decision should be based on what works best for your child and fits your individual belief system. In general, a newborn baby will eat 2 to 3 ounces of breast milk or formula a day for every pound of body weight. So a 7-pound baby may require 14 ounces or more of food each day. In the beginning your baby may eat more frequently, but a routine gap of 3 to 4 hours is healthy as your baby ages. As you become more adept at the feeding process, each feeding might last from 15 to 30 minutes. These numbers are basic guidelines. If your baby is wetting a normal number of diapers each day and gaining weight, you are probably doing a fine job. Your physician will monitor your progress and answer any questions you have.

Burping

Every baby must be burped. The frequency with which burping is needed depends on how much air your baby swallows while feeding. Babies with a larger palate cleft often require more frequent burping because they have a tendency to swallow more air. Watch your child for cues as to whether or not he needs to be burped. He may stop feeding, begin to fidget or fuss, or slow his sucking rhythm. To burp your baby, hold him upright—either on your shoulder or in a sitting position—or lay him across your lap. Pat and rub his back gently until you elicit a burp, being sure to always support his head. You might have to do this several times during a feeding or only once when the feeding is over.

Cleaning Your Baby's Mouth

Think of your baby's mouth as being similar to a self-cleaning oven: you really should not have to do anything to clean it. If, however, you notice some milk curds or bits of cereal in the cleft area, offer your child a few swallows of water to wash the area clean. If this does not work, you may wipe the area with a clean, damp cloth. NEVER use a swab or syringe to clean your baby's mouth; they may cause injury.

Blaise Winter, National Football League Player, Writer, and Speaker

Born with a unilateral cleft lip and palate, Winter found himself facing adversity at a young age. After discovering football, Winter found the acceptance he had always craved.

Playing for the Indianapolis Colts, Winter was named to the NFL's First Team All-Rookie list. He continued in the NFL playing for the Green Bay Packers and the San Diego Chargers. He ended his career with a damaged knee, standing on the sidelines as his team vied for a Super Bowl Championship. (They lost to the San Francisco 49ers.)

Winter's first book, A Reason to Believe, *describes growing up with a cleft palate and his experiences in the NFL. Winter is now a motivational speaker whose work has brought hope to thousands of people.*

Introducing Solid Foods

Some groups believe that food should be introduced at a specific age; others, when your baby reaches a certain weight. As you would with any healthy infant, take your cues from your child and the advice of your physician. In general, solid foods can be introduced when your baby is between 4 and 6 months old.

Begin with a rice-based cereal mixed with breast milk or formula so that it is quite thin. Sit your baby in an upright position (this will help with possible nasal regurgitation). Using a spoon, not a bottle, place a small amount of the cereal on your baby's tongue. Do not be alarmed if your baby sucks at the food, causing some of it to regurgitate through her nose. Eventually, with practice, your baby will be able to move the food to the back of her mouth. Also do not be alarmed if your baby gags on the food; this is a new experience for her. Do watch her carefully, however, so that she does not choke.

As your baby becomes more adept at eating, you can introduce other strained foods. It is recommended that you introduce one type of food at a time in order to watch for any reactions from your child, such as allergies or food preferences. Eventually you can introduce "melting" foods such as ring-shaped cereal and saltine crackers. Avoid anything sharp, such as chips and nuts. Your child will learn to overcome the sucking instinct and begin to chew the food. As each new food is introduced, your child will explore the new texture and taste. You may see a temporary increase in nasal regurgitation. This is perfectly normal. If your child is having trouble eating solid food, contact your physician team for advice.

The American Cleft Palate Association recommends the following as a guideline for introducing solid food. This is only a guideline—you should consult the professionals who oversee your child's care for individualized advice.

4–6 months: Introduce cereals and pureed foods.

8 months: Give liquids, pureed foods, ground or junior foods, and mashed table foods.

12 months: Give liquids and coarsely chopped table foods, including most easily chewed meats.

18 months: Give liquids and coarsely chopped table foods, including most meats and many raw vegetables.

(Source: *Feeding an Infant with a Cleft,* p.18, 1997)

Your baby may have very few feeding differences from any other child. Unless the cleft presentation is severe, you can follow almost any medical feeding chart.

Eating Utensils

As your child grows older and more independent, he or she will want to take over more aspects of self-care, the first of which is generally feeding oneself. In the beginning, your baby will use a pincher reflex to grasp finger foods from the tray of a high chair. As he becomes more adept at fine motor skills, he will want to use a spoon, fork, and cup.

Introducing a cup can be a wonderfully comic experience. Your baby will explore the device by turning it upside down. Once he discovers that the liquid will drip, he will make a game of emptying the cup and playing in the liquid! A sipping cup with a spill-proof lid may help circumvent this problem. Help your child with the first few attempts at sips. Lift the cup to your child's lips and allow some of the liquid to enter his mouth. You may demonstrate drinking with your own cup. Once you have modeled the proper behavior, allow your child time to experiment on his own. To introduce spoons and forks to your child, use smaller, safer utensils manufactured specifically for children. Some spoons have a soft-coated bowl, ideal for the beginner. There may be a problem with your child's using silverware during the recovery time after surgery. Watch her carefully if the palate has not completely healed. It is rare for a child to poke silverware through the newly reconstructed roof of the mouth, but it has happened. Using a straw can be learned once the muscles of the soft palate are strong enough. Sucking on a straw is a great way to exercise these muscles. Try not to let your child become frustrated if this skill takes time to master—it takes time with all children, whether they had a cleft or not.

Pacifiers

Your situation, your belief system, and your baby are all unique. The decision to use a pacifier is dependent on all three. Again, there are groups that will recommend against using one and there are groups that will recommend its usage. Pacifiers are great for exercising the sucking response and strengthening the muscles of the soft palate. Some children who cannot suck enjoy "gumming" the pacifier. Some babies with a cleft prefer having nothing in their mouth. It is recommended, however, that you limit the use of a pacifier and end it altogether before it can affect the placement of teeth, or if it may have an adverse effect on a surgical repair.

In Conclusion

The most important factor in your child's nutrition and feeding habits is you. Communicate with professionals when you have questions or concerns, and use your own knowledge of what works best for your baby and your situation. This will form a solid basis for making decisions about feeding. If your baby is eating healthful food, gaining weight, and has healthy body functions, you are to be congratulated.

CHAPTER 4

Coping with the Emotional Impact

Having a baby with a cleft palate, especially if you were not fore-warned about the condition, can be an emotional experience. You may feel a mixture of emotions ranging from joy and happiness to fear and doubt, even anger and guilt. You may even feel guilty about your feelings! This roller coaster of emotions is normal. You are not insane. You are simply reacting to the trauma of having a baby who is not exactly what you had planned.

You need time to grieve the loss of the "perfect" baby of whom you dreamed as you planned for this birth. A healthy grieving process means allowing yourself to have these feelings and deal-ing with them. It also means acknowledging that fact that these emotions will resurface from time to time as surgeries or check-ups approach. This, too, is normal. This chapter aims to help you understand and embrace a myriad of emotions—all of which are legitimate and necessary for you to grow stronger and more healthy.

Counselors and Confidants

We are by nature social creatures. It is normal for you to seek out friends and family members with whom you can share your emotions and dreams for your child. It is important to find people who will listen to you without ridiculing you or shutting you down. If you cannot share these intimate emotions with your spouse or significant other (who, you must remember, is wrestling with a variety of emotions just as you are), seek out a trusted friend or pastor. There are mental health agencies and counselors readily available in virtually every area. They may be found in the yellow pages of any phone book. Referral services can help you find a counselor or agency in your area.

Seeing a counselor no longer carries the stigma of old. It does not mean that there is something wrong with you. Rather, seeing a counselor is generally a wise and healthy response to painful circumstances. A good counselor can help you focus your grief and walk you through it so that you can come to a healthy acceptance of your situation.

Finding the right counselor may involve interviewing or meeting a few different people until you find someone with whom you feel comfortable. Do not be afraid to ask questions. Find out if the counselor supports your belief system. Any counselor with whom you feel uncomfortable may not be the person best suited to help you. Whomever you choose to confide in, be sure that you know you can express yourself without the fear of being judged. If you find your friend or counselor giving you advice and solutions when you simply need a sounding board, tell her so in a gentle, considerate manner.

Support groups may be available in your area or at a nearby hospital that houses a craniofacial team. The American Cleft Palate Association, a local referral agency, or your local pediatrician may have information on one of these groups. If no group exists and you feel the desire to form one, leave word at local doctors' offices, in church bulletins, and at hospitals. Forming a support group is discussed in Appendix C.

Journaling can be the safest confidant of all. You can vent your feelings, give words to your fears, use language you would never utter aloud, and then close the book. Sometimes getting things down on paper on your own can be just as helpful as seeing a counselor.

Shock

The sight of a cleft-affected child may shock you, especially if the lip is affected. That pearly little pout you expected may not exist. Instead you may see a parted lip, extended gum tissue, or missing pieces of your child's face or mouth. The shocked, numb feeling is normal. In fact, it may help to sustain you in the first few days, insulating you from strong emotions and allowing you to function. You must be careful, however, not to use this numbing insulator to suppress your emotions completely. Eventually, in order to be a healthy and functioning parent to your child, you must face and experience your emotions.

Take a moment to look at your child. Familiarize yourself with his facial defects. They are a part of your baby. And they can be repaired! Now look carefully at his eyes. Touch his soft head. See your child's beautiful traits. Count his fingers and toes. Touch his chubby belly. Cradle his little smooth bottom. This is your baby. The cleft is such a small part of him. As Joanne Green once stated, "This is a baby, not a cleft."

As you become accustomed to the face of your child, your shock will diminish. As you learn more about the wonderful medical advances that will help your child lead a rich and fulfilling life, your pain will ease. In fact, many parents experience a new sense of grief after lip adhesion surgery: they miss the double smile their child used to have! The baby with the completed lip looks like their child, but there is a slight difference. It may take some time to get used to your baby's new look.

Other people may be as shocked as you were at the sight of your child. If you have other children, prepare them for the sight of their new sibling by sending home a picture from the hospital. Have someone explain the cleft to them in their own language. Perhaps they can be told that the baby has a "broken lip" or that the baby's lip didn't finish growing. Then be sure to point out that the doctors will be able to fix it in time.

Allow your other children to visit the baby as soon as possible. Allow them to ask questions about the baby's cleft presentation. Answer the questions as thoroughly as possible in a calm, matter-of-fact tone. If you aren't sure of an answer, tell your child you will ask the doctor. Try not to express any negativity toward the baby. If you accept this baby, whether perfect or slightly flawed, your children will accept him. Your calm attitude and proper preparation will help your children get past their own shock.

The same methods may be used in explaining the cleft to adults. A picture, a brief explanation of the cleft, and assurance that the cleft can be repaired is sufficient. If you do not feel comfortable calling and telling others, have your spouse or significant other, or a trusted friend, do the calling. Don't forget to emphasize that you have had a baby…who just happens to have a cleft palate.

Kurt Dykhuizen, Child Actor

You may not recognize the name of this young actor, but you will recognize the show on which he played. Dykhuizen portrayed the character of Jason on "Barney and Friends." The show, which championed diversity, used children from various ethnic and cultural backgrounds as well as those with various levels of ability.

Guilt

As we discussed earlier in this book, guilt is often a natural first reaction to giving birth to a baby with a defect. We wonder what we may have done to cause the defect. We wonder if we are being "punished" in some manner for wrongs done in our past. We wonder if we somehow don't deserve to have a "perfect" baby. We may even begin to feel guilty about our feelings toward the baby. How could a "good" mother not be overjoyed at the birth of her child? We may tell ourselves that the negative feelings we have, including anger or sadness, prove that we are "bad" parents. In a self-perpetuating cycle, we then may begin to feel guilty about our own emotions and guilt!

Once again it must be emphatically stated that *this is not your fault!* This precious child you hold is a gift to be celebrated. The flaw is a minor part of that child. It will not keep your child from laughing and loving and living. You did not harm your child. In fact, you will be the person most instrumental in repairing that physical flaw and helping your child build a healthy, self-assured personality. Your love, acceptance, and nurturing will have a far greater impact on your child than a small physical defect.

Your baby has been born with a defect, a flaw. But isn't every human being in existence flawed? When put in perspective, a physical flaw may be more desirable than a broken or malicious spirit. Your job is to work with the team of surgeons and therapists to help your child progress through a series of reconstructive surgeries while building her self-esteem and confidence. If you are feeling a strong sense of failure or responsibility, talk this over with a counselor or trusted advisor. Sometimes the process of admitting a sense of guilt may help to eliminate it.

Fear

Fear is one of the first emotions to overwhelm the new parents of a cleft-affected child. Along with the emotion ride the questions: Can this be fixed? Will our child be normal? Can our child learn to speak? How will we afford surgeries? Where do we find help? Education is your best ally in laying to rest your fear and answering your questions. You have already taken a strong step forward in this direction by obtaining this book. You may find more information on the Internet or in the local library. Speak with people who have "been there," whether as parents or as people born with a cleft. Talk to members of the craniofacial team. Ask questions and do not stop until they have been answered. The more you know about the many options available to you and your child, the less fearful you will become. In general, fear is bred in a spirit of darkness and ignorance. Do everything in your power to overcome that ignorance both in your household and in those who come into contact with your child.

Grief

It is normal to grieve the loss of something you hold precious. The dream of the baby you planned for has not been lost, but perhaps altered. It is okay to grieve the loss of the images you held. It is healthy, too, to weep over the struggles you and your baby will face. This is an unfortunate turn of events, something you did not plan on or choose. Grief is vital if you are to accept and recover from the loss you have been dealt. Allow yourself the time to cry. Your sadness is genuine.

Don't allow anyone to tell you that you should "get over it" or, worse, try to shame you for your valid emotions. The person who tells you that you should not be sad because your baby is healthy is doing you a disservice. While it is true you can celebrate a healthy baby, you have also been dealt a painful blow. You cannot simply wish your feelings of loss away, any more than you can wish away the cleft in your baby's mouth.

While grieving generally progresses through certain stages, the process is personal. There is no single way to grieve, just as there is no steadfast time limit on grief. We also know that once you have passed through one stage of grief, it may return at another time. Some of these stages can also occur at the same time. Or you may never experience some of them at all. Each person is different. If you find yourself stranded in one of the stages or unable to cope with daily life, it is strongly recommended that you seek help from a professional counselor. Even if the grief you are encountering is less traumatic, having a trained individual to help you through this time of loss and pain can be beneficial.

In general, the stages of grief include a time of shock or numbness during which you may not feel anything. You may then begin to feel guilt and sadness over your loss. This may be followed by disbelief or a yearning for the time before the birth of your baby when things were still "okay." You may find yourself fantasizing about your baby having a perfect little mouth. During this time you may find it difficult to concentrate, relax, or sleep. You may enter next into a bargaining phase, in which you make promises to God or a Higher Power on the condition that they "fix" your baby.

You may feel strong emotions of anger, sadness, and depression. You may have outbursts, yell at others, become snappish or easily irritated. You may burst into tears without warning. And you may begin to withdraw from those around you, especially close friends or family members who have "perfect" babies. As you work through these feelings and begin to find methods of coping, the sadness will become less sharp, the depression will lessen. Eventually, you will come to a place of acceptance.

Unfortunately, just as you are hitting some of the most volatile stages of grief (usually 4 to 7 months AFTER the loss), your friends and family members may push you to "get over it" and get on with your life. In today's society we have a tendency to gloss over the grieving process and rush through it. Rushing through your grief or bottling it up inside will cause repercussions later in the form of emotional problems or physical illness. Take each stage a step at a time, seeking help as you feel is necessary.

Depression

Many women experience post-partum depression after the birth of their baby. This may be caused by the hormonal changes occurring in their bodies. It can be compounded by the exertion of giving birth and the exhaustion caused by caring for a new infant. The "baby blues" can occur in varying degrees of severity. Sleep, a good cry, and the passing of time help most women overcome this depression; for some, however, medication and counseling are recommended.

Add to this your sadness over your baby's cleft and you could swing into a serious depression. Sadness is a normal part of the grieving process; it is only when sadness consumes you that it may become dangerous. If depression lingers or is severe, you must seek help both for your sake and for the sake of the infant who needs you. A depression that leaves you unable to function is not just the "blues"; it is a serious medical condition that can be alleviated. Speak with a counselor about ways to cope with your depression.

Michael Berryman, Actor

Born with Ectodermal Dysplasia, Michael Berryman had no fingernails or fingertips, no hair, no sweat glands, no teeth, calloused skin, and a cleft palate when he first came into the world. Berryman overcame the odds to play roles in many films. In a career spanning more than two decades, he has appeared in One Flew Over the Cuckoo's Nest, Doc Savage, Star Trek 4: The Search for Spock, *and* The Crow. *Berryman also spends time speaking at symposiums for various organizations, including Wide Smiles.*

Confusion: What If I Don't Know What I Am Feeling?

Life is never black or white, emotions are never cleanly delineated. You may feel a rush of various emotions all at once. Other times you may feel...nothing. Sometimes one powerful emotion will come to the fore, only to be replaced by another, even stronger emotion. You may find yourself laughing and crying at the same time. Again, this is normal. Dealing with mood swings is a part of everyday life in our fast-paced society. You do not need to spend your time analyzing and labeling every emotion you feel—sometimes it is okay simply to feel them, acknowledge them, and move on. However, it may not be healthy to minimize or trivialize continued mood swings. If your emotions are moving too rapidly and you feel out of control, professional counseling can help you get a firm grasp on them.

Sometimes it helps to identify a pattern in your moods. Sometimes these emotions may be hinged on outside cues such as a specific scent or sound that reminds you of the first moment you saw your baby, or the place where you heard someone speak unkindly of your baby's face. Rather than withdraw from these physical cues, realize what they are and try to superimpose another thought on them. Always remind yourself that the emotional upheaval you feel is a natural part of moving through grief to health and acceptance.

The Toughest Question: Why?

We may seek an answer to the ultimate question for a lifetime and never be satisfied. Or we may be able to see the tangible fruit of having a cleft-affected child. Our belief system may tell us that our baby is a reward, a test, a method to strengthen us, or simply a sweet baby to love and nurture. This baby is not a punishment or a burden. The cleft your child carries is not a mark of shame, nor is it something horrible or unforgivable. It is simply a cleft. It can, and will, be repaired.

In time, we will be able to leave the open-ended question of "why?" and move on without concrete answers. Bad things happen even to the best people and we cannot always know why. Your baby does not deserve a cleft, nor does he deserve the surgeries and therapies in his future. But they are a part of our flawed world. They are a reality for your baby and your family. Be angry with the fact that this world is imperfect, but do not be angry at the innocent child you hold, and do not be angry at yourself.

Allow the "why?" in your life to come alongside a "why not?" Why not receive this wonderful child who will enliven your home and enrich your lives? Why not enjoy the sweetness of your child, the laughter and silly antics he will bring? Why not accept the gift of this beautiful child with a very slight defect? Why not rejoice even as you face the sometimes-painful future?

A Crisis of Faith

The birth of a child with a cleft may rock, if not shatter, your belief system or faith. One of the most difficult causes of guilt can be the hidden anger we hold toward the God or Higher Power in whom we believe. Many of us were taught never to question God, let alone be angry with God! The guilt our anger produces may become a dark secret, left to fester and damage our spiritual life. Before you let that happen, consider this: If the Higher Power in which you believe is truly powerful, isn't that Power great enough to hear your anger? If you believe your God is all knowing, doesn't that same God already know you are angry?

Take a walk, go for a drive, or write a letter and talk to your Higher Power. Tell of your fears, your sadness, your anger. Rant and yell and cry. Share your heart in words or song. You will not be deemed a "bad person"...just a human being with frailties and emotions. (The Judeo-Christian God actually invites people to wrestle with difficult issues and even with God himself. In Chapter 32 of Genesis, we see Jacob, the father of the Israelites, wrestle all night with God and receive a blessing. In this text, there is an invitation to "wrestle" out our issues with God and ask him to bless us.) Talking to your Higher Power about your anger is a healthy method of wrestling with and understanding your own belief system. You may also want to seek out a priest, minister, rabbi, or other spiritual leader to help you find answers in your crisis of faith.

You may find that family and friends fall back on religious clichés when discussing the birth of your cleft-affected child. You may hear "It's God's will," or "God only tests those who have a strong faith," or "God won't give you more than you can handle," or, even worse, "There are a lot of people who have it even worse than you do!" Before you blow up in anger, take a moment to consider the motivations of the person speaking. Isn't it true that, inept or painful as his words may be, he is sincerely trying to help you? If you take a moment, you may find some grains of truth in his words that will help to sustain you.

Joy: Celebrating Your Baby

No matter what emotions you may be feeling, be sure to celebrate the birth of your child. A new baby is a reason to rejoice!

Announce the birth of your child, receive congratulations, and then mention the cleft. There are many ways to celebrate the wonderful new addition to your family: hang a welcoming banner in the front window or in your work area, order a yard sign, or place an announcement in the newspaper. Send out announcements—either with or without pictures, depending on how you feel. Have a party. Invite friends to donate to a cleft palate organization such as About Face or The American Cleft Palate Association in your baby's name.

Treat this baby as you would a baby born without a cleft. Fill out a baby book and continue to record milestones in your baby's life. Take pictures—not just clinical or documentary pictures that will show the progress of her reconstructive surgery, but portraits and candid photographs. These pictures will show that you love and value your child just the way she came to you, that your love is not dependent on a perfect mouth. Allow yourself time to grieve, give voice to your feelings and fears, dream about the future, and celebrate the wonderful new baby you hold.

CHAPTER 5

A Word to Families and Friends

You are in a unique position to help the new parents of a cleft-affected child. Your unconditional support and friendship are vital to help them through the healing process. Accept that these parents have suffered a painful loss—the loss of the "perfect" baby of whom they dreamed and for whom they planned. The reality of having a child with a birth defect may throw these parents into a whirlwind of emotions. They may feel adrift, afraid, and unsure. You are in a position to be a rock for them, as a sounding board, a helper, and a friend.

That Important Initial Reaction

You may not have met the baby yet. If this is the case, prepare yourself for the sight of a cleft lip, which can be a bit disturbing for some. Look over the pictures in this book. Peruse the photo gallery on the Wide Smiles website. Educate yourself on clefting and its reconstruction. Go over the earlier chapters of this book.

When you enter the room and greet your friends, the first and most important thing you can do is congratulate them on the birth of their new child. This is a reason to celebrate! If you are comfortable, ask to hold the baby. Comment on the beauty of the baby. Does she have big, round eyes? Does he have a lot of hair? Are her cheeks puffy and pink? Is his skin rich in color? There are a myriad good qualities on which you can comment.

Admire the baby first, but do not ignore the cleft lip or palate. You may have seen a photo essay of a baby with a similar cleft who now looks wonderful—tell the parents about it. Share positive stories you have heard of children who speak perfectly after reconstructive surgery, therapy, or both. If you have no stories to share, simply tell them you are concerned and that you think their baby is beautiful. A big hug will speak volumes to the family. Do not be afraid to cry with them in their season of pain— knowing that you care will be healing for them.

What NOT to Say

* Try to avoid speaking in clichés or brushing off a parent's legitimate concern. Don't tell parents that "everything will be fine, don't worry." Everything may not be fine for a long while. And any loving parent is going to have many times of worry as he raises his child.

* Some people feel that they must say something, anything, and end up blurting out hurtful things without meaning to do so. If you cannot think of anything to say, that is all right. Your presence tells the parents you care.

* Avoid telling parents "horror stories" about other babies with birth defects. The new parents do not want to hear worst-case scenarios of other babies born with clefts. Don't mention a distant cousin who has a profound hearing loss that is blamed on his having a cleft palate left unrepaired for too long. Don't assume that, by hearing the plight of children worse off than their own baby, the parents will feel better. This baby is their reality. It is their "worst-case scenario." Don't try to shame them into saying that it isn't as bad as something else.

* Don't nickname the baby or make fun of the cleft. As much as you may want to joke and lighten the mood in the room,

the baby or the situation should never be the target of your humor.

* Don't compare the baby to other famous disfigured characters such as the Elephant Man or Quasimodo. Neither of these had a cleft lip or palate. The fictional Quasimodo is a wonderful lesson in not judging someone's heart by his outer appearance. You may be guilty of doing just that when you label the cleft-affected baby with these names.

* Try not to gasp or back away when you first see the baby's face. Take a moment and consider the entire face: the eyes, the nose, the hair, the cheeks. The cleft will become less and less prominent when seen in proper perspective.

* Do not tell the parents that they must have done something to cause their baby to have a cleft. They are feeling enough pain and guilt without having someone they care about make accusations.

* Do not try to be an expert and tell the parents everything they should do to care for this baby. Unless you are a physician, avoid giving them your prognosis and advice for reconstructive surgeries, speech therapy, or other areas of development that are best left to the professionals.

* Weigh your words carefully. They can never be unsaid.

What If My Foot Is Already in My Mouth?

Did you already have an adverse reaction to the baby? Have you already said something you regret, something that may have hurt the new parents? By all means, apologize for any pain you may have caused. Write a note or pay a visit to the parents. Explain that you were shocked or frightened or simply made a bad attempt at lightening the mood. Tell them that you realize what you have done and that you are sorry. Let them know you value their friendship and are concerned about them. Go on to tell them something wonderful about their baby and congratulate them on the birth. Make every effort to repair the damage done to your relationship. These parents need a strong support network during this time, as surgeries approach.

Showing Your Concern and Support

There are many ways in which you can show your concern. Sometimes a simple visit can help a stressed parent through a rough day. As a more tangible means of showing your support, give the new parents a gift or card congratulating them on the birth of the baby. Don't mention the cleft or express sympathy. Just give a standard "Congratulations on the New Addition" type of card, or a typical baby gift: an outfit, a blanket, a plaque, a toy. Treat the birth of this baby as you would any other.

On a separate occasion you may wish to send a brief note or card of encouragement. Tell the parents you are thinking of them as they struggle through a difficult time. Let them know you are there for them. You might even include a gift with this card, such as a coupon for a lawn or diaper service or a month's worth of maid service. Something that can lighten the load will be appreciated. Be sure to make these two very different expressions of love and concern two separate events. Don't combine them.

Becoming a Sounding Board

Parents of a cleft-affected baby will react in various ways. Some will become quiet and withdraw. Others will display an almost obsessive need to talk about the baby and the cleft presentation. In either instance, you have an opportunity to help your friend come to terms with the whirlwind of emotions that accompany the birth of this baby. Your physical presence and willingness to listen are vital assets.

The parent who is withdrawn may find comfort in simply sitting together with you to watch television or go fishing. If your attempts to get her to talk about the baby or the situation are rebuffed, allow her to stay quiet. The talker may seek you out as a sounding board. He may need to think things through by saying them aloud. Do not be too eager to jump in with advice. Many times the talker is not seeking advice at all. He may simply need someone to listen with a nonjudgmental attitude.

Acknowledge and validate the parent's feelings. Don't tell him you know how he feels unless you have a child who was born with a cleft. Tell him you can see how frightening it must be or how it might make one angry or sad. Ask him how something he relates made him feel. Help him to explore the complexity of his emotions by giving voice to them.

Do not tell her that she is wrong to feel the way she does. Give her sympathy and tell her that feelings are never right or wrong; only actions may be judged by that standard. Assure her that wrestling with emotions is a normal part of the grieving process. If your desire is to "fix" the situation, try to realize that by simply listening, you may be doing more to "fix" it than by giving advice. Finally, if your friend seems depressed or is having trouble functioning, encourage her to see a counselor to help her through the shock and grief that she is experiencing.

Bernice Brooks Bergen, Model and Actress

This beautiful woman, born with a cleft, made her dreams come true by becoming a professional model. She is proof that no matter the social stereotypes, there is room for beauty that is not absolutely "perfect."

Ways You Can Help Around the House

Having a new baby around the house can be exhausting. First the mother needs to recover from the process of giving birth, then she may be nursing a baby around the clock. The father may be bottle-feeding and changing diapers. Both of them are losing sleep, and probably worried about the welfare of their child. Add to this the pressure of having a baby with a birth defect, the assorted visits to specialists and doctors, learning to feed a baby who cannot suck, and many other fatiguing activities. Something has to give—and you are in a perfect position to help the parents let go. You can do any of the following on your own, or speak to others and gather a small army to battle on behalf of your friends.

* Offer to pick up the older children and take them to your home for an afternoon or overnight. Give the parents time to be with their littlest addition without the worry of neglecting the others.

* Offer to sit with the newborn for an hour or two while the parents leave for a cup of coffee or a long walk...or a nap. If the baby has recently been fed, assure the parents that you can watch and cuddle the baby for a short while.

* Bring over a hot meal. Organize others to bring meals. Keep a chart and have one hot meal brought to the house every night or every other night in disposable containers. This frees the parents from having to plan a meal, shop for it, and then clean up afterward. As any parent of a newborn knows, those plans can be interrupted at any time...for a long time! Disposable containers allow the parents to eat and be free of the drudgery of clean up. They can focus their energy on meeting the special needs of their child.

* Pop in for a housecleaning. Bring along a friend and make a day of it. Wash the floor, dust, sweep away cobwebs, wash windows, scrub the bathroom, vacuum. Make the house shine. The gratitude you see on the faces of your friends will swell your heart.

* Help out with the laundry and ironing. Offer to do it there, or pick it up and take it home. Return a basket full of freshly pressed clothing. Don't forget the sheets!

* Bring over a can of gasoline and get the lawn mower out. Trim hedges, edge sidewalks, weed a garden, shovel snow, de-

ice the walk. There are so many chores to be done around the house, and the new parents probably cannot get to all of them.

* Run errands, shop for groceries, and ferry older children to lessons or activities. If you enjoy driving your car, these types of jobs can be fun as well as rewarding.

* Gather up a collection from other friends and help replace a broken screen door, or have concrete delivered for that broken patio slab. Help erect a play-yard fence. Replace that faulty water heater or any other broken item your friends have been complaining about.

Gathering Information

* With their hands full caring for a special-needs child, the new parents may not have time to seek out information at libraries or on the Internet. You can do this for them. Research clefting websites and print out information, or check out books for the family.

* Talk to professionals you may know. Ask them about clefting and reconstructive surgery, as well as speech therapy and other factors in the development of a cleft-affected child.

* Contact local support groups through your local pediatrician or hospital. Find out where and when they meet and then offer to drive your friend to a meeting. Or watch the baby while your friend attends.

* If it's possible, and the new parents do not mind, make contact with someone who was born with a cleft and arrange for him or her to speak to the parents.

* If there are no support groups in the area, and the parents are interested in forming one, help them. Use Appendix C of this book as a guide.

* Consult your friends' insurance policy (with their permission)

and determine what coverage is offered for the various procedures and equipment needed for the baby.

* Help the parents obtain the necessary letters from professionals if coverage is denied.

* As a last resort, contact the Insurance Commissioner for your state to find out what can be done to help the baby receive the care she needs.

* If you write well, offer to draft letters for your friends.

* Contact state and federal aid programs to find out criteria for grants or aid for the parents and the child. Many agencies will help with the cost of equipment or medical care.

* Help parents plan for each hospital visit if the hospital is out of town. Help with transportation, baby-sitting older siblings, or arranging housing.

* Make yourself available in whatever capacity you feel comfortable. Use your gifts and talents to ease the burden of the new parents.

Helping to Educate Others

* A trusted friend or family member may be just the person to prepare older siblings for their first visit to the hospital after the baby is born. Take a picture of the baby along with you and explain the cleft to the children in simple terms (see Chapter 4).

* If you live in a small neighborhood, you may take the first step in alerting the neighborhood to the birth of the baby. Explain that the parents will be rejoicing and grieving at the same time. Show them pictures of cleft-affected children. Encourage them to visit the Wide Smiles website.

* Affirm that the baby is healthy and is not in pain. Suggest that the neighbors read this chapter, or paraphrase it for them.

* Take some time to carefully explain the baby's cleft to the children of the neighborhood. Assure everyone that the cleft can be repaired.

* Organize the neighbors and make a "Welcome Baby" banner. Have everyone sign it. While you're organizing, have the neighbors sign up to do some of the tasks and errands listed under "Concrete Helps in the Home" above.

* Offer to contact extended family for the new parents. Announce the birth of the child and carefully explain the cleft presentation. Assure them the baby is fine but will need reconstructive surgery. Helping to educate others will save parents the job of having to explain and reexplain their situation.

An Opportunity for the Church or Synagogue

It can be difficult to know what to say to parents who have a healthy baby with a cleft lip or palate. Follow the suggestions outlined in "That Important Initial Reaction" above. First, congratulate the parents on the blessing they have received. Find the good in this gift of a child. Admire the baby. And then sympathize with the family. One church announced the birth of a child, allowing the congregation to applaud and celebrate. Later in the service the congregation was asked to pray for the baby's well-being. It was in the second announcement that the cleft was mentioned, not the first.

Do send someone to the hospital to pray and be with the parents. Sitting alone in a hospital room with your fears is extremely difficult. Organize a prayer chain on behalf of the parents and the child. Pray that the baby will be healthy, that the correct craniofacial team will be located, that the parents will find comfort and strength. Send the parents a note telling them that dozens (or hundreds or thousands) of people are praying for them. Be careful not to use religious jargon or clichés to smother the parents' need to mourn the loss of their "perfect" baby. Allow them to express that grief. Support them and remind them of the love and comfort readily available to them through their church or synagogue... and through their God.

Senator and Mrs. John McCain

Senator McCain and his wife, Bridget, adopted a little girl who had been born with a cleft palate. Their daughter, of Asian descent, is thriving in the loving care of these special parents.

After the Initial Crisis

As the baby grows, surgeries and therapies will have to be undergone. Stay in touch with the parents. Revisit "Concrete Helps in the Home," send cards, visit the hospital, organize friends and neighbors, and bring meals in during recovery (the parents will have their hands full with their child after surgery). Continue to reach out to the parents as they revisit their original grief or mourn something that has just come to light. Your love and unconditional support may be one of the most important factors in helping the new parents cope with the difficulties of raising a cleft-affected child.

CHAPTER 6

Dental and Orthodontic Issues

Many craniofacial teams include two or more specialists in dental work. Your child may be treated by a dentist, an orthodontist, and a prosthodontist, if dental prosthesis devices are necessary. Each has a vital role in the treatment of your child's cleft presentation. While orthodontic treatment such as braces seem to focus on achieving "good looks," it is actually a vital part of ensuring proper speech placement and better oral health.

The Dentist

Like any other child, your child should begin regular dental hygiene as soon as the first tooth erupts. Swabbing teeth with a damp, clean cloth after meals, teaching your child to brush and floss, and visiting a dentist are critical for good oral health. Because your child is seen by a team of physicians on a regular basis, he may visit a dentist earlier than many children. Generally, a child will begin dental visits at approximately age three. Until that time, the parents are responsible for teaching his good habits in oral hygiene.

During the first visit to a dentist, your child may have X rays taken of her mouth to study tooth placement and check for cavities or irregularities. These films might not be taken until the child is older, however, if there is no evidence of a problem. Your child may need to see a dentist if a tooth erupts in an unusual place inside the mouth. This sometimes happens if tooth buds were moved during surgical procedures on the palate. If the tooth is not causing a problem with speech or eating, it can be left in place. However, if a tooth that is out of correct position causes problems, it may be removed by the dentist. Often this will occur during palate surgery.

The dentist will instruct you as to proper methods for cleaning your child's teeth and gums. This may be a bit more involved than with other children if some of your child's teeth are in unusual positions. Your child may enjoy using a battery-powered or electric toothbrush. Some speech therapists encourage their use in order to stimulate the alveolar ridge and help enhance the health of tissue and its response to various stimuli. It is a fact that improper care of the baby teeth can have a negative impact on the health and development of the permanent teeth, jawbone, and facial bones. Losing a tooth may affect not only the speech of your child, but also the ability of the orthodontist or prosthodontist to attach devices to the teeth. Any concerns you have about dental hygiene should be addressed to the dentist on the cleft palate team or to the plastic surgeon acting as head of the team.

Special Dental Care for Cleft-Affected Mouths

While it is best to see the dentist on the cleft palate team, local dentists and specialists also may be effective in treating and maintaining your child's oral health. You should ask any dentist or specialist you plan to use whether she has experience working with children with cleft presentations. You should also question her about her willingness to work with your child's cleft palate team.

The dentist should be aware of the unique issues involved in dental work for cleft-affected children. Often these children will begin orthodontic or prosthetic work at a much younger age than other children. They may be missing some teeth, have teeth that are turned, or sprout teeth inside the cleft or on the palate. Some of the teeth may be shaped incorrectly. A child with a palate or gum cleft may have improper *occlusion* (the relationship of the upper teeth to the lower teeth), or may require a device or appliance to widen the palatal arch. In some cases, teeth are removed to facilitate growth, placement, speech or other factors. Some of this work may begin before the child has any permanent teeth. If the baby teeth are in proper position, it is easier for the permanent teeth to be guided into position.

The Prosthodontist

A *prosthodontist* is a specialist who works by augmenting existing mouth structure with obturators, bridges, or dentures. An obturator is a plate that is used to complete closure of the palate. It can help stop air leakage through any opening or fistula in the palate that could directly affect speech development. It can also help reduce nasality. The obturator may act as a retainer during palate expansion or as a bridge to supply missing teeth. It also may be used before surgery occurs in order to facilitate feeding. It may be used in place of some surgeries when there is insufficient tissue to repair a cleft or the child is not healthy enough for a surgical procedure—or it may be used in conjunction with surgeries to produce optimal results. Your child's team will advise you as to whether or not an obturator is recommended for your child.

Depending on your child's unique cleft presentation, he or she may be missing some teeth. This problem can be remedied with dentures or bridges or even implants. You should be aware, however, that as your child grows, the dentures or bridges will probably need to be replaced.

The Orthodontist

Orthodontic work includes the realignment or repositioning of teeth, correction of irregularities, palatal expansion, and revision of crossbites (a presentation in which the upper teeth are inside the lower teeth). Children as young as 3 or 4 years old may begin some of the early work with an orthodontist. It is critical that you use an orthodontist who has experience in working with cleft-affected children. The work done by this specialist can affect not only speech and appearance, but it can also impact the midfacial growth and any bone grafting in the alveolar ridge area. An aggressive orthodontist may not be the best person to treat your child. Be sure the work is in alignment with the overall plan of the cleft palate team, whose continual monitoring will aid the orthodontist in the timing of bite plates, expanders, or braces.

Orthodontic treatment varies with each unique presentation. The length of treatment, the devices and appliances used, and the use of prosthetic devices are all determined by your child's cleft. Some children require the use of a palate expansion device. This device attaches to the teeth on each side of the upper jaw. You will be taught how to turn a small screw that will in turn push the upper teeth and jaw out over the lower jaw. The expansion that takes place is a slow process and produces little discomfort. Your dedication to following the orthodontist's procedural outline will have a direct impact on the length of time the expansion device must be used.

If your child has a cleft in the alveolar ridge area, orthodontic treatment may be used as preparation for bone grafting. If this is the case, be sure to follow instructions and the time line you are given carefully. Overly aggressive work on this area of the mouth can result in graft rejection or *midfacial retrusion* (a condition in which the middle of the face does not grow at the same rate as the rest of the face, resulting in a flattened or concave profile) in rare instances. If you are concerned about this possibility, discuss it with the team leader.

As each new treatment begins, your child may feel some discomfort as she gets used to the adjustments. Each appointment may bring additional adjustments that cause tenderness or discomfort. The discomfort is short-lived, however, and should be gone within a few days. The orthodontist might recommend soft foods and soups for a day or two, making a successful visit a great excuse for ice cream!

After completion of treatment, your child may be fitted with a retainer. A retainer is generally removable and fits over the teeth and palate. The retainer may include false teeth if your child has any missing teeth. It may be used indefinitely or until a permanent bridge or implant is completed. Remind your child that the retainer keeps her teeth from moving back into a former position. Not wearing the retainer can result in the need for further orthodontic work. Remember, the success of your child's treatment lies not only in competent dentists and orthodontists, but in cooperation from you and your child as well. Do not skip appointments, follow directions, and observe good oral hygiene.

Jan Johnston—Horse Whisperer

Johnston trains and schools horses using the methods featured in the Robert Redford film The Horse Whisperer. *Her interests and involvements include a leadership role in her church, raising her two daughters, and riding her horses. She has been known to take time out of her busy schedule to reach out to new mothers of children born with a cleft lip or palate.*

Braces and Mouth Guards: Getting Through the Teen Years

As your child reaches his teen years, the need to look nice often becomes more important to him than proper speech or medical factors involving a cleft. Encourage your child to focus on the end results of orthodontic and prosthetic work: a beautiful smile, self-confidence, better speech, and a healthy life. With braces becoming more commonplace, your child will be "one of the crowd" while wearing them. And the attractive smile that will result goes a long way in convincing a teenager that others find him desirable as a friend or romantic interest. Allow him some ownership in the plan for his teeth by including him in the team meetings whenever advisable. Give him some choices, but help him to understand that some decisions are yours...and are non-negotiable.

If your child is active in athletics, discuss the chosen sport with the orthodontist. Often, if the sport involves contact, a mouth guard of soft plastic may be used to protect the teeth. Most cleft palate teams encourage involvement in activities, with consideration given to unique situations such as a recent surgery. Treatment may last years and should not hinder a child from participating in activities with his friends. You can help your child get through the long months of treatment by promising a special reward when the braces come off. You might consider a vacation, a special gift, or a new privilege.

CHAPTER 7

Helping Your Child to Cope

Communicating with Your Child

Answering Questions

As your child grows, he will begin to ask about the world around him. Questions such as "Why is the sky blue?" or "Where does the moon go during the day?" will almost certainly come around to "Why do I have a scar on my lip?" or "Why did God make me different?" The best answers are honest and nonjudgmental. If you do not know an answer, tell your child the truth. Then suggest that the two of you search for the answer together. Page through this book with your child, search the Internet, contact The American Cleft Palate Association, speak with one of the members of the child's cleft palate team, visit a library. Spending this time with your child will demonstrate to him that you place value on his need for answers. It shows him that he has dignity and worth and will build his self-esteem as few other actions can.

As you discuss your child's cleft, explain that there was nothing she did to cause it. She is not being punished for anything. She is not bad. Let her know that you love her and will help her to be the very best person she can be, and that a cleft will have no bearing on that. Explain to your child that you do not like having to see her hurt or have surgeries, but that you know the outcome will far outweigh the difficulty of the present time. Tell her that your decisions are always made with her best interests and future in mind.

Allow your child to question you about every aspect of his care and habilitation. Answer his questions concisely and honestly in language he can understand. Allow him to have input in some decisions. Be firm with your child when some steps in the treatment are deemed necessary, but allow him some leeway in decisions that are not as critical. Keep him updated on upcoming procedures; *never* surprise him with treatments or surgeries. Preparation and ownership are critical in helping your child cope. Also, provide your child with a safe environment for venting anger or sadness over his situation. It is normal for your child to be angry. After all, he did not ask to be born with a cleft. Why shouldn't he be resentful over the pain and tedium of treatment and therapy?

Validating Your Child's Feelings

Above all, do not hush a child who wants to talk about her feelings. Our instincts may tell us to brush away fears and anger with a calming "It will be fine. Don't worry." But this does nothing to relieve those emotions. It simply teaches your child to hold them inside—which can have a devastating impact later on her emotional maturity. Allow your child to express her feelings, and listen carefully to them. Then validate the feelings, whether or not your agree with them. Repeat what your child has told you in your own words. For example, after listening to your child vent about how ugly the scar makes her feel, you could say, "What I hear you saying is that you are angry about having a scar on your lip. Is that right?" Allow her to answer. Or you might say, "You must feel really angry about having that scar. What do you think we can do to help you with that anger?"

Validating a child's emotions, not brushing them aside, will help your child feel open to discussing those feelings with you. Never tell a child that his feelings about the cleft are "wrong." Feelings and emotions are never wrong; they just "are." Explain this to your child, telling him that we have choices about how to react to our feelings. Our actions can be deemed right or wrong when seen in the context of social, moral, and religious beliefs. For instance, you may talk about how angry your child feels after being teased about his scar. Tell him you understand how hurt and angry the teasing must have made him feel, then explore various actions that may be taken. Should your child hit the person doing the teasing? Should he find something about which he can tease the other child? Should he ask for peer mediation at school in order to explain to the other child the reason for the scar? Should he ignore the teasing? Discuss each option, and help your child decide on a course of action. Help him to see that the emotion behind the actions is the same in each case, but the action may be right or wrong depending on your social, moral, or religious values. In following this process of validation, brainstorming solutions, discussion, and deciding a course of action, you are teaching your child a vital life skill while showing love and acceptance.

Time for Venting

There may be times when your child loses her temper. Allow her a safe environment while holding to the boundaries set within your household. You may even give your child a time limit on venting in a certain manner or assign a certain "rule-free" venting area. For example, if your child has just found out about an unexpected complication and is seething with anger and fear, you may suggest a 10-minute venting time in her bedroom. Together, set some guidelines: there will be a 10-minute time limit; any words may be used without punishment (including or excluding profanity); things may be thrown but not broken; pillows may be hit; the door must be closed (or open). Set a timer and allow your child the freedom to "get it all out." Afterward, hold her... cry together...talk...and assure her of your love and support.

The Psychologist or Social Worker on the Team

As your child ages and becomes more aware of the world around her, as well as how she fits into that world, the psychologist on the craniofacial team will become more of an asset. This trained and licensed individual will help you and your child find solutions for the potential emotional impact of scars and future surgeries. If the hospital or clinic that houses your team is some distance from your home, the psychologist or social worker may also be able to refer you to counselors in your area who specialize in working with children or who have experience working with cleft-affected families. Speak with the team psychologist or social worker if you suspect your child is having a difficult time accepting the cleft, is having social problems, or seems overly quiet, angry, or sad.

Jeff Peggs, Lawyer and Head of a Mentoring Camp for Children

Not one to rest on his own achievements as a lawyer, Peggs established a Nebraska-based "cleft camp" that builds the self-esteem of cleft-affected children by showing them first-hand what a person born with a cleft can achieve in life.

Other Venues for Counseling

Private counseling is a boon to many children. Some start in the elementary grades while others don't begin until they reach the teen years. Some find counseling unnecessary. It must be stated that the social taboos about seeing a counselor or psychologist that were prevalent years ago are a rarity now. There is nothing wrong with seeking the help of someone who can help restore us to health. We do not hesitate to see a doctor if our child is physically ill; we should not hesitate to see a counselor if our child is unwell emotionally. It would be a rare child who did not struggle with some aspect of being born with a birth defect that requires surgeries and therapies over the course of several years. If your child is having trouble adjusting, is acting out at school, or is threatening to harm himself, you may not be able to give him a choice over whether or not to see a counselor. In these cases, you may have to tell him that a counselor is a requirement right now.

Finding the right counselor for your child may take some time. Ask the cleft palate team for suggestions. Others who may advise you include school counselors, teachers, or religious leaders whose opinions you trust. Taking into consideration your personal belief system is important, since a child may become confused by having a counselor who gives advice that is contradictory to the family's religion or beliefs. Some spiritual leaders themselves make wonderful counselors. The only caution here is that they may be untrained in certain areas of counsel pertaining to the physical flaw. You must carefully weigh the benefit of spiritual counsel against any areas in which it may be lacking.

Once you find a potential counselor, help your child come up with a list of questions for the counselor. Arrange a meeting during which you and your child may ask these questions. Allow your child to speak freely to the counselor. Do not be insulted if your child or the counselor requests time for the two of them to speak alone. After the first meeting, ask your child how he felt about the counselor, allowing him to speak freely. Together, you may then decide if this counselor will work out for him. When your child has begun seeing a counselor, do not press him to share details of the sessions with you. Allow him the privacy and respect he deserves. Listen carefully if he decides to share information with you, and avoid making judgmental statements. Encourage him to continue to be honest and open with the counselor. Never tease your child or make jokes pertaining to counseling, and do not allow his siblings to do so. Stress that counseling is an important part of becoming a healthy individual.

Creative Expression

There are many ways of expressing emotion. Some of these may not seem to pertain directly to the cause of emotions, but can help to focus them in a positive manner. Help your child find the methods that most appeal to her, allowing her opportunities for creativity and honest expression. Encourage her to use a journal to write down her feelings and experiences. Decide with her whether the journal will be private or something she can share with you or another trusted adult. Journals may be used in various ways. Perhaps your child can use it to write a record of her feelings and experiences. Or it may be used to write fictional stories in which the heroine has a problem similar to your child's. Allow your child to use the journal in any manner she chooses.

Writing and the Fine Arts

Creative writing such as fictional stories or poetry can help a child express and explore emotions without personalizing them. It can be a "safe" way in which to brainstorm various solutions or put ownership to thoughts that may cause him to feel guilty. For example, your child's poetry may speak of hatred and pain, allowing him to vent on paper. Teenagers often find that venting their angst helps them to cope with the complex emotions common to their stage in life. Don't punish a child for the language and images used in poetry—you may, however, ask him to discuss the poetry with you or with a counselor. If your child is writing about violent acts such as harming himself or others, it should be brought to the attention of his counselor or the psychologist on the cleft palate team. Threats of suicide or violence should always be taken seriously. Be sure to tell your child that you are acting out of concern and deep love.

The fine arts are a wonderful venue for expression. Piano lessons, painting classes, dance classes, and other activities allow your child opportunities for success and enjoyment while teaching discipline and the acquisition of a lifelong skill. When helping your child explore artistic possibilities, keep in mind anything that may be hindered by the cleft presentation. For example, a child with a severe bilateral cleft may wish to consider percussion lessons rather than flute when joining band. (The presentation of the cleft may make focusing air properly for the flute quite difficult.) A child who has great difficulty with speech might consider singing lessons with a studio that emphasizes personal growth and skill rather than performance or competition. Discuss various options with your child honestly and gently. She may choose to pursue a difficult performance option against the odds. Once the decision is made, do all you can to support and encourage her in her chosen venue.

Athletics

Just as valuable as the arts are athletics. They, too, allow for individual growth and expression, as well as lessons in sportsmanship and discipline. Help your child test various sports during the year. He will eventually settle on those that he most enjoys. Giving him the opportunity to choose his sport is allowing him another step toward independence. Be sure to communicate with a coach or instructor if a procedure or surgery may affect an upcoming event. Obviously, your child will have to sit out any activity that may injure a newly reconstructed gum line or have a negative impact on a lip revision. Outside of those rare occasions, allow your child to simply be "one of the team."

Commitment Times

Encourage your child to try as many venues as she wishes. It is wise, however, to establish a "season" rule: "Try any sport or class. If you do not like it, you may choose not to pursue it in the future, but you must finish out the season without quitting."

Discuss this rule with your child before the start of the season or class (with lessons you may set a time limit of one year or one school year) so that she understands it before making a decision. This rule teaches your child perseverance, dedication, and commitment. She learns to stick with something even when she is not fully enjoying it—for the benefit of herself and her teammates. Some children even find that the activity they despised becomes one they love before the season is over. This and other lessons make the value of the arts and sports in a child's growth inestimable. The benefits will be reaped for years to come in terms of self-esteem, character development, stability, and friendship.

Psychosocial Problems

Many children battle feelings of inferiority, and a child with a scar on his face or difficulty speaking may be especially prone to such feelings. Help your child understand that everyone is flawed in some way, but that everyone has something to offer. Go over your child's class roster. Have him point out something each child can do better than he can *and* something he can do better than each child. For example: "Jimmy can jump higher than I can, but I can spell better than Jimmy." Discuss the fact that everyone has something they do better than another. Jumping higher does not make Jimmy a better person. Neither does spelling better make your child better than Jimmy. Many children with a speech problem develop a fear of speaking. This may be compounded by teasing in school. Spend time practicing therapy exercises with your child. Stay in close contact with his speech therapist. Help your child to develop speech skills that will enable him to be clearly understood. Praise successes no matter how small they may be. Encourage your child to join in on dinner conversation. Try to avoid answering others for your child. Allow him freedom of expression, and do not criticize any attempts he makes. Never embarrass your child by correcting him in public; instead, offer help in a private setting.

Many children born with a cleft lip or palate become self-conscious or shy. This may be due, in part, to the reaction of others. It may also have some roots in the attitude of the members of the child's family. If you behave toward the cleft scars as though they are horrible reminders of a terrible defect, your child will absorb that attitude. If you treat the scars as a very minor part of a wonderful kid, your child will absorb that attitude. Your child's siblings should be taught to treat not just your cleft-affected child, but each other as well, with dignity and respect. If your child is teased at school, help him or her to express the emotions the situation causes. Discuss the type of child that teases. Could it be that the teasing child has some insecurities of her own? Could she be trying to impress someone?

Discuss the total effect the cleft has on your child. Does being born with a cleft make him less of a person? Does it make her less intelligent? Is a really big part of who your child is? Help your child to see all the wonderful aspects of his personality, gifts, talents, intelligence, and appearance. Is he a good friend to others? Does she help children who struggle in school? Is she friendly? Does he have a great sense of humor? Affirm each positive quality. Your attitude toward your child will go a long way in helping her develop a healthy respect for herself and others.

Michael Christy, Baby Beauty Contest Winner

Proving that being born with a bilateral cleft lip does not prevent a child from being beautiful, Michael Christy has won trophies in baby beauty contests and was crowned "Prince of Lancaster."

Helping to Make "Different" Become "Special"

Many schools make a point of teaching diversity and tolerance courses. We are becoming a nation more attuned to the value of diversity in education and community. Parents hold a sacred responsibility to teach our children acceptance and tolerance of others, as well as to encourage respect and healthy curiosity toward cultures different from our own. You may spend some time teaching your child about the various subcultures that make up our rich heritage in the United States, drawing his attention to the fact that all people are different. Point out that every person has something to contribute to society.

Make a trip to the public library and check out books on different cultures and minority groups. Read biographies of important minority figures such as Martin Luther King, Jr., and Willie Mays. Read about the vast diversity of Native American cultures and traditions. Ask local museums or educational groups about art shows, storytellers, musical performances, or festivals that celebrate different ethnic groups. Introduce your children to a variety of people. Help her to understand and accept people of other religions and belief systems. Read about the traditions celebrated by those groups. Your acceptance of others will have a great impact on your child's ability to accept them, and to see her own value as well.

As you discuss the value and contributions of each cultural or religious group, steer the conversation toward people who have made contributions to our society—and the world at large—who had disabilities. Explore and share the biographies scattered throughout this book that detail the accomplishments of many cleft-affected people. Seek out information on other people who have made the best of their lives despite their disabilities. For example, Albert Einstein had a learning disability...and yet became one of the most brilliant scientists of the 21st century. Composer Ludwig von Beethoven wrote some of his best music while completely deaf (check out a CD of his Ninth Symphony and play it for your child, explaining that Beethoven himself never heard this music). Troy Aikman, legendary quarterback of the Dallas Cowboys, was born with a condition called clubfoot and required surgeries. Recording artist and Academy Award–winning actress Cher has a learning disability, as does actor Tom Cruise. A bit of research on the Internet or in the library will reveal dozens of successful people from all walks of life who were born with a disability of some type. Help your child see that a disability does not hold a person back from making a great impact on the world.

Educating Others

As your child begins interacting with others, she may find for the first time that her cleft has become an issue. Where once no one mentioned it unless there was a doctor's visit or therapy scheduled, she may now find others teasing her or frightened. Discuss this possibility with your child—it may be best to do so before she begins school. You may begin by telling her that sometimes children are frightened by something they do not understand. Explain that her cleft might cause another child to be afraid. Tell her how to help the other child understand and accept the cleft scars or the remaining cleft in a gum line or palate.

Practice with your child by discussing possible scenarios. Ask him open-ended questions such as "What do you think you could do when someone teases you about your cleft or your speech?" Help him to brainstorm answers that involve educating the other child. Help him to see that retaliation in the form of anger, physical violence, or one-upmanship ("I may have a cleft, but you're stupid...and I can have my cleft fixed!") is never a good option. It may make your child feel better at the time, but in the long run he will find that cruelty and mean-spirited comebacks only cause more problems, both socially and individually.

By using Appendix A in the back of this book, you can help your child's classmates and teachers to understand more about clefting. Ask your child's teacher to speak frankly with the class about clefting. Once young children understand a disability or difference in a classmate, they are usually very accepting. Still, have the teacher watch for teasing in the classroom, and discuss the attitudes of the other children with your child. It is critical that you keep the lines of communication open with her. Always offer your support and love. Whenever possible, allow your child to handle any social problems at school. Help her to come up with solutions that she can then implement.

It is appropriate to remain in contact with teachers and guidance counselors concerning these issues. Unless the problems become severe or continue for a length of time, try to keep your communications with educators private. If a teasing situation becomes chronic, if your child begins to fear returning to school, or if he develops headaches or stomachaches, speak with counselors and teachers and decide on an intervention plan. Remember, you are your child's advocate in all areas of health. This includes emotional health and social contacts. Cruel treatment should never be tolerated, and every effort should be made to help him overcome such treatment while teaching other children tolerance and acceptance. If the school must intervene, stress the importance of mediation rather than punishment for the offending parties. It is best to mend relationships rather than permanently destroy them. If a mediation session with your child and the other party does not cause a cessation in the teasing, it may be wise to switch one of the children to another class. School counselors are trained to deal with these situations; work with the counselor to find the best solutions for your child.

CHAPTER 8

Speech and Hearing

It is quite possible that your child has already been assigned a speech therapist through your county's Early Intervention or Birth to Three program. Although it may seem odd to have a speech therapist work with an infant, you will reap great benefits from the expertise of this professional. During the infant stage, the therapist will assist you in overcoming any feeding issues that may arise. In time, the games the therapist plays with your child will develop the pre-verbal skills necessary for speech and language to begin. The therapist may even teach you and your baby some basic sign language, to help you and your pre-verbal child communicate, and will teach certain skills in listening, speech, and language that will help your child become intelligible.

As your child ages, the Early Intervention program may offer classes and language groups that will help her to use her new skills in experiences with other children and adults. The program may also provide periodic testing not only in speech development, but also in large-muscle motor skills, fine motor skills, and cognitive ability. The therapists on the cleft palate team will work in conjunction with the county therapist to find the best possible strategies. The speech therapists will also work with the team ENT, or *otolaryngologist*—a specialist concerned with the function of the ears, nose, and throat. The ENT will test your child for hearing problems, place tubes if they are needed, and work with you to overcome any hearing loss.

The Ears

As previously mentioned, children with soft palate clefts seem much more susceptible to ear infections. This condition, if chronic, may necessitate the implantation of ear tubes similar to those used for other children with recurring ear infections. The procedure is generally done under general anesthetic and in conjunction with an early surgery such as lip or soft palate reconstruction. A small hole is placed in the eardrum, and a tube (generally shaped like a T) is then inserted in the hole (with the upper cross bar placed inside the ear). You may notice some blood or drainage for a day or two after the insertion of the tubes. This is perfectly normal. The ENT will instruct you on caring for the new tubes as the ears heal. This usually consists of placing drops in the ears for a number of days. Caring for the ears after that time will involve wearing earplugs during certain activities such as bathing; soapy water may cause the tubes to slip. Ask the ENT for any specific precautions that should be taken.

Before the tubes are inserted, your child's doctors may treat ear infections with antibiotics. Once the tubes are in place, you will usually be able to spot an ear infection because there will be evidence of drainage. The infection can be treated with a combination of antibiotics and eardrops. At times, the tubes may become blocked by earwax or matter that drains from inside the ear. If a tube becomes blocked, the ENT may prescribe drops. In rare instances, the ENT may have to open the tube or replace it altogether. Your child will continue to have ear checks with each visit to the cleft palate clinic.

Audiology

When your child begins attending the cleft palate clinic team check-ups, he will begin having hearing tests. These will be continued on a regular basis for years. You might sit in a room with the audiologist and your child. Your cooperation and ability to sit quietly without drawing his attention will greatly aid the outcome of the test. Various sounds will be played and your child's reaction recorded. Eventually, he will be asked to look in the direction of the sounds or to perform a task when a sound is played. These early tests are not completely accurate: they may be used to detect some hearing loss, but they will not indicate which ear is not fully functional.

Another early test, which will be repeated at various stages of your child's development, is the *tympanogram*. This measures pressure on the eardrums and can help detect fluid in the eardrums, blocked tubes, and potential hearing loss. As your child becomes more verbal and able to understand and obey directions, he may begin to be tested wearing headphones. This allows the audiologist to test each ear individually and watch for hearing loss at various frequencies. A beep or noise will be played over one side of the headset. He will be asked to raise the hand on that side or look in a specific direction when he hears the tone or noise. While hearing loss is rare among cleft-affected children, it can occur. Early diagnosis and treatment, including hearing aids and therapies, will help him to develop language more readily and function with fewer difficulties.

Shayne Stillar, State Champion Bicyclist

Shayne Stillar was born with the congenital condition identified as Aperts Syndrome. He had an underdeveloped midfacial area and anomalies of his hands and feet. Stillar underwent reconstructive surgeries at the University of Minnesota. In 1995, Stillar won the Minnesota State Time Trial Championship for Category 5 Stock Division. He believes that with hard work, anything is possible.

Speech Development

Language development consists of a number of sequential stages. It must be remembered that, as with children who are not cleft-affected, these stages vary according to the development of the individual child. The first stage in a child's development of speech and language skills is the *instinctive* or *reflexive* stage, during which infants utter sounds and vocalizations based on their needs. Hunger, fatigue, distress, and other factors compel the child to grunt, cry, or make noises. The sounds have no meaning in themselves but are merely instinctive. When a baby reaches about 1 month in age, the sounds change and become more isolated and unique. He is able to respond to various feelings or stimuli with a variety of beginning sounds. This stage will develop into a *babbling* stage in approximately the third month. During the babbling stage, your baby will coo and gurgle, respond to your facial expressions and voice, and be able to differentiate among his own responses.

Between 6 to 8 months, babies begin to play with and repeat the sounds they enjoy making. It is not unusual for a child in this stage to squeal and giggle over her own attempts at making noises. Before long, the baby will begin to imitate the sounds she hears. It is important in this stage to talk and sing to your baby. The more verbal interaction you have with her, the faster language is developed. Next your child will enter the *linguistic* phase of development, during which actual words are learned and repeated. It is important to speak to your child in adult speech patterns rather than baby talk so that correct learning takes place. Your child will begin the linguistic phase by using a sound or single word to represent something specific. Eventually verbs and adjectives will appear in sentence-like phrases. The final stage is reached with complete sentences and the continued development of vocabulary.

Encourage your child's efforts in each of these stages with warmth and smiles. Negative reactions could impact her attempts at speech therapy. Correct your child gently by giving the proper pronunciation of a word. Realize that the normal development of speech does take some time, even for children without a cleft.

Sign Language

Pre-verbal children may be able to learn rudimentary sign language in order to facilitate communication with their parents and siblings. Simple signs for *please* (rubbing a hand in a circle on the chest area), *more* (bringing the fingertips of both hands together in a horizontal position), and *eat* (bringing the fingertips of one hand to the mouth as though lifting food) can help your child make herself understood. You may want to consider learning a few more signs than this; studies have shown that children who learn sign language while pre-verbal learn language at a faster rate. And a physical movement combined with a spoken word helps children to remember the new word more easily.

Sounds and Phonetics

Generally, by the age of 3, a child will have mastered most of the vowels and combined vowel sounds. He will also be able to pronounce consonants such as *p/b*, *m*, *w*, *t/d*, *n*, and *h*. His vocabulary should be approximately 800–1,000 words. A child with a palatial cleft may have some trouble with the voiced and unvoiced consonants: *p/b* and *t/d*. These consonant pairs are produced in a like manner, with one consonant in the pair using more vocalization than the other. By approximately 5 years old, a child with an alveolar ridge or hard palate cleft may still struggle with blended consonants such as *bl*, *br*, *pl*, and *st*. However, he should be quite intelligible and have added *k*, *g*, *f*, and *v* to his vocabulary. A soft palate cleft may prevent the clean articulation of *k* and *g*, while an alveolar cleft may affect *f* and *v*. Beginning at age 6, but sometimes a bit later, children will begin to master the *s*, *z*, *sh*, *ch*, *tch*, *zh*, *l*, and *r* sounds.

Cleft-Affected Speech

A child with a cleft lip or palate may experience delays in the stages of speech development. Your child's speech therapist will work with you and your child by practicing techniques that will help her produce the proper sound placement. At first the therapist will appear to be simply playing with your child. However, this "play" will facilitate both trust and a comfort level that allows the therapist to introduce new sounds without the child even becoming aware of the learning experience. Eventually, the speech therapy may become more focused on isolated sounds. The therapist may give you drills to use with your child that repeat the targeted sound. This will, in turn, develop into using the sound at the beginning or ends of words. Finally, your child will be encouraged to use the sound in complete sentences.

It is normal for a child to master a sound in isolation and then lose the sound when using it in a word or sentence. For example, a child may be able to make a perfect *v* sound when saying it alone. That same child may then say "I bacuumed the carpet" when asked to use the sound in a sentence. Therapy will help your child become more consistent in using sounds. Sometimes your child may reach a point where speech development halts until another surgery or procedure is performed. The speech therapist and the team will work with you to plan a course of action if this is the case.

Sean Mundy, Child Soloist

It is always an honor to be selected as a soloist in a choir, but for a child born with a cleft lip and palate resulting in speech delays, the honor is also a victory. Little Sean Mundy was asked to solo in the Grades 3–5 Spring Concert at his school. He sang "Gary, Indiana," from The Music Man.

The Parental Role in Speech Development

Your role in your child's speech development is critical. You are the primary teacher. You need not be an expert in speech and language, nor do you have to go over vocal drills and exercises for hours and hours. Your first task is to interact and talk to your baby. Verbalize whenever possible: explain the diapering process, go over the grocery list, describe things you see on a car ride. The more language your child hears, the more she can absorb.

Sing to your child. You do not have to have a trained singing voice... or even a good singing voice. Your child loves you and your voice is one of her favorite sounds. Not only is singing a wonderful way to bond; it has also been proven that music is a great way to learn. Children retain more information when it is set to music. And children involved in music have tested as having higher-level math skills, longer attention spans, and high ACT scores. Sing to your baby. Sing with your child.

Give your baby a treat and imitate the sounds he initiates. Follow your baby's lead. This game becomes a precursor to your child's imitation of your sounds. As your child enters the linguistic stage, continue talking to him as often as possible. Encourage your child to try to pronounce new words. It sometimes is best to avoid asking, "Can you say...?" Often the answer back will be "no." Instead, try saying, "Let's try this new word. I bet you can say it pretty well."

When working on sound development using speech drills, be sure your child can see your mouth clearly and that you can see his. You may also give your child a hand mirror to hold so that he can watch his own mouth while attempting to imitate you. Ask the speech therapist for games or exercises you can play that target the goals and sounds you and the team have determined need work. You might find it beneficial to actually purchase a few of the toys and books you see the therapist using. You may then copy the techniques used by the therapist. Picture books and plastic animals are great for helping your child learn to make animal noises and say animal names. A photo album or scrapbook is an excellent tool for teaching a child to say the names of family members and friends. Make up silly sentences and gibberish words using targeted sounds. Help your child to say as many words as he or she can think of using the isolated sounds.

Above all, be sure that your child attends therapy sessions and any language groups. Work with her speech therapist and ENT to ensure that she is learning proper technique and placement for sound. If additional surgery is advised to facilitate speech, discuss it with the cleft palate team. Work with the therapist before and after the surgery in order to continue a structured and cohesive speech and language plan for your child. Remember that every child, whether cleft affected or not, develops speech and language at an individual rate. Expect more delays if your child's cleft presentation is severe. Be patient and diligent with her, celebrating each victory as it is achieved. Your confidence in her will translate into gains in self-esteem and perseverance. You are your child's most important asset in speech and language development.

CHAPTER 9

Financial Considerations and Concerns

One of the more frightening aspects of medical care can be the costs. As technology advances, costs increase due to a number of factors. Training specialists is expensive. The equipment used for various tests and procedures continues to be improved. New inventions and techniques continue to come to the fore, as research continues to enhance the outcomes of the procedures used. Each of these advances is exciting and holds promise for your child—however, they also cost money. Some insurance policies cover most, if not all of the expenses incurred in the treatment of a cleft-affected child. Some have co-pay programs. Others have worked out contracts with participating clinics and hospitals to curb costs by using specified fee limits.

If your child is not covered by an insurance policy, or your policy is inadequate to cover the costs incurred in treatment, there are some other options available to you. You may qualify for Medicaid, charitable funds, grants, or programs in which physicians donate their services. Some organizations donate or help cover medical care if you can provide your own transportation to a particular hospital or clinic. Another option available, although more time-consuming and difficult, is fund-raising to cover the costs of treatment.

Insurance

Take the time to review your policy. You may have either a group or an individual plan. The policy will state what is covered and whether or not you are limited to a certain group of physicians, clinics, or hospitals. It will list any co-pay plan, deductible (dollar amount you must pay before the company begins payment), and coverage limits for the family or individuals. Some policies will include a lifetime limit on moneys spent by the company. A stop-loss limit sets an annual limit after which you will no longer have to pay for a specified service. If you have any questions about coverage and deductibles, contact your insurance agent or the insurance representative at your place of employment. You may also contact the insurance company itself with any questions by calling the number listed on your insurance card or in your policy handbook. Prepare your questions and have them in writing before contacting a representative. This allows for efficient use of time and may aid in your being taken seriously. Take careful notes during your conversation. Ask for clarification on any point you do not understand. It is wise to ask for some promised coverage in writing if it is not specifically listed in your policy.

Health Maintenance Organizations (HMOs) and Preferred Provider Organizations (PPOs) may specify a fixed rate set by a group of physicians, clinics, or hospitals. You may be liable for a certain portion of some costs. Generally, an HMO will have a limited list of providers from which you must choose. You may also have to have a written referral for every visit to your specialists. PPOs, on the other hand, may allow more freedom of choice, with reduced costs when you use their preferred providers. Traditional insurance plans may hold you liable for a part of the health care costs after a deductible has been met. You may have more discretion in selecting a physician, clinic, or hospital.

When Insurance Does Not Pay

At times, you may receive a denial of services. This may be questioned and your claim resubmitted if the service, equipment, or procedure was deemed necessary by the team in charge of your child's care. Sometimes denial of coverage may be the result of a misunderstanding and, once the problem is addressed, coverage may be instituted. For example, an insurance company may deny coverage of lip adhesion surgery because it is considered cosmetic. A letter from a team representative explaining the treatment, the reasons for it, and the outcome may be necessary to convince the carrier to pay for the procedure. Dental work during cleft surgery is sometimes denied by medical insurance. You may need a letter explaining the necessity of extracting a tooth that had erupted in the hard palate, causing a fistula. Sometimes procedures may cross over from one type of coverage to another. Some medical equipment that is normally not covered may be covered once the company understands the medical necessity of its use. For example, a breast pump may not be covered for the mother of a healthy nursing child, but may be covered for the mother of a child whose cleft will not allow the child to nurse.

Carefully consider any denial of coverage, question its validity, and, if necessary, pursue the matter. When contacting an insurance company, it is best to follow the "chain of command." Begin with your agent or insurance representative at work. They can help you formulate a letter or tell you what papers should be collected and submitted. If you are still not satisfied with the service you receive from the representative, contact the company directly. Do not be afraid to ask to speak with a claims supervisor. Follow any telephone conversation with a letter. Be sure to state: "...according to our telephone conversation on (date) at (time), you informed me that...." Once all avenues at the company have been tried, and if you and the team find that a company is unrightful in denying coverage, it is perfectly acceptable to contact the state insurance commissioner. If coverage is still denied, do pay what you owe.

Medicaid, Welfare, and Other Charitable Organizations

If you do not have insurance coverage, or your coverage is inadequate, you may qualify for Medicaid or other social aid. Contact your local Birth to Three program, county health organization, welfare agency, or social services agency to apply for aid. Your physician, clinic, or hospital may put you in touch with these agencies. They are also listed in the local telephone book under the "Government" heading. AboutFace, Operation Smile, and others may be contacted online. The Cleft Palate Association is a wonderful resource for agencies that help children with cleft lip or palate. Rotary, Elks, Lions, Optimist, and other service clubs in your area also may be willing to help.

Each of these agencies will tell you specifically what is required to qualify for aid. Most require a proof of residency, birth certificate, and/or social security card. A worksheet is generally used to determine eligibility, with questions on family income, assets, and resources; the number of dependents in the household; the parents' marital status; and/or proof of the parents' employment or unemployment. Some charitable organizations ask for copies of unpaid medical bills or letters from the cleft palate team. Others require that surgeries and therapies take place in a sponsored hospital or clinic. Be aware that some organizations and grant programs limit their funding to children with terminal conditions or lasting disabilities. Because clefts can often be repaired, giving them the status of a "temporary" disability, these organizations will not aid a cleft-affected child

Meghan McCartney, Figure Skater

Meghan McCartney and her sister, Shana, competed together, at the ages of 10 and 7, in the Ice Crystals Figure Skating Competition in New York. Both sisters won medals; Meghan, who was born with a unilateral cleft, won the silver.

Fund-Raising

Some counties allow families to raise money for medical expenses by holding fund-raising events; some require a license for such events. You must check with your local government in order to proceed legally with medical fund-raising. Once the way is cleared for a fund-raising event, contact friends and family members who may be interested in helping organize it. Other groups may also be interested. Churches, high school business clubs, or volunteer organizations may be willing to provide the manual labor involved in such an undertaking. When you have your core group of volunteers, decide on the type of event. Raffles, dances, concerts, contests, and dinners are all means to raise money. You can even combine more than one type of fund-raiser. You might have a dance with a raffle or a dinner with an auction.

Contact local businesses or service organizations and enlist their aid. Some may donate goods or services for a raffle, while others may donate help. Local high school students may donate services such as lawn mowing or snow shoveling for a raffle; mothers may donate baby-sitting services. Brainstorm ideas with your core group. Do not forget to contact local athletic and arts organizations. Most professional teams, community theaters, and other groups will donate tickets, signed items, or posters to charity fundraisers. Some music groups, speakers, or athletes will make an appearance and waive their usual fee if the cause is something they feel is important. Keep in mind that if you don't ask, you won't receive.

As you contact each group or organization, have a photograph of your child ready. Keep a list of estimated procedures and their costs. You can even show the group a breakdown of the cost of your child's most recent procedure. Explain where the insurance shortfall lies. Some of the people you contact may prefer to give a cash donation. Others may decline to become involved.

Whether you receive a donation of goods, services, or money or you are turned away, maintain a polite and professional demeanor. Thank the person for his or her time. Your attitude may make a difference if you have to raise funds again in the future.

When Money Is Short

Remember that the hospital is not the "bad guy." They are not trying to "stick it to you" with exorbitant costs. They have simply provided a service that is expensive. It costs them money to have the latest technologies and specialists available for your child's care. If you find that you are truly unable to meet the costs, contact the financial office of the physician, clinic, or hospital. The representative will meet with you to come up with a plan for payment. They may require many of the same papers as the charitable organizations discussed above. They may also require a proof of debts owed to other institutions. The hospital or clinic will try hard to make a plan that will work for you. After all, receiving some money in small payments over time is far better than receiving nothing.

A final and more drastic option is to declare bankruptcy. Before taking such a step, contact a financial planning organization or lawyer and discuss your options. Bankruptcy will have a far-reaching impact on your life and future finances and credit ratings.

Financial Planning and Budgets

Many families find that having a child with medical needs places a strain on the household finances. Adopting a workable budget will help ease that strain. Financial planners are available in most larger communities. You can hire a consultant for a fee or contact a charitable group such as Catholic Social Services, Lutheran Brotherhood, or FISC (Financial Information Service Center). These groups are listed in the telephone book under "Finances," "Financial Planning," or "Financial Consultants." Be prepared to track your expenditures for a few weeks, provide financial documentation, and work out a budgeting worksheet of fixed and variable expenses. Once a budget has been planned, hold to it religiously. If, in a few months, you find that the plan does not work for your family, meet again with the consultant. Go over the plan and brainstorm ideas for adapting it to your family's lifestyle.

Simplification and Lifestyle Changes

Some families try to simplify their lifestyle when faced with the costs of treatment for a cleft-affected child. There are literally dozens of books on this subject. Check your local library for titles. Simplifying may include such minor changes as taking a shorter vacation, purchasing generic products rather than name brands, or canceling a cable television subscription. Involve your entire family in coming up with a plan for simplification. Your children may have clever and innovative suggestions, and are more likely to follow a plan that they have had a hand in developing. Allow each person to be as creative as possible in the brainstorming session. Do not ridicule any ideas—simply write them down and discuss them. You could allow a family vote on some of the ideas.

Some family members may be willing to scale back on expenses and donate the money to a medical/therapy fund. Try walking or biking to work or school instead of using the car. Hang clothing on a clothesline in nice weather to avoid running the dryer. Turn the thermostat down two or three degrees. Quit smoking. Institute a family game or activity night instead of going out for fast food or a movie. With a little ingenuity and commitment, your family can find the means to help your child receive the care he needs to become a healthy, productive adult.

CHAPTER 10

Aiden:
One Child's Story

I hadn't expected this pregnancy, although I had hoped for another child eventually. We already had two boys and two girls, the youngest of whom was only four months old. In fact, I was still nursing my little girl full-time and hadn't even started menses after my pregnancy with her. I had just turned 34 and on most days had barely enough energy to keep up with my brood. But for days I just hadn't felt right. I picked up a home pregnancy test while grocery shopping one morning. It was a bright fall day so I treated the children to a backyard picnic for lunch. While they were eating, I slipped into the house and took the test.

Positive. I clutched the test in my hand and stood in the doorway watching my children. They chattered happily, the baby cooed in her infant chair. Looking down at the test in my hand, I began to feel faint. The edges of my vision grew hazy. The chatter of the children became muted, as though I were underwater and far away from them. I shook my head, willing myself to remain calm. In an instant I was able to accept this reality: I was having another baby. Suddenly I felt excited, sure that the new baby would be as wonderful as the other children. And I began to look forward to its birth.

The pregnancy went well. There was a touch of nausea in the first trimester, but it was fleeting. In fact, I felt better than I had during any of my previous pregnancies. I was, however, exhausted by the end of each day. Keeping up with four children under the age of 6 took more energy than I had! Several weeks into the pregnancy, I submitted to some standard tests that screened for certain birth defects. I'd had these tests with each child and did not anticipate any problems until the obstetrician called. Although he could not be positive, the test indicated a high chance that this child might have Down's Syndrome, a congenital disorder in which one chromosome is doubled. The condition can include mental impairment, a flattened skull, shortened leg bones, and almond-shaped eyes. The doctor recommended an ultrasound test, explaining that he could measure the leg bones and make some general conclusions about the likelihood of the baby's having Down's Syndrome. Another test, an amniocentesis, would give conclusive results.

Amniocentesis involves inserting a needle through the woman's abdomen and into the uterus. Amniotic fluid is drawn. Cells in the fluid that are sloughed from the baby are then genetically tested. A printout of each chromosome is made. If the 21st chromosome is doubled, Down's Syndrome is diagnosed. Amniocentesis is not without risk: there is a chance that the test will result in miscarriage. However, a mother can wait to have the test until the baby is viable, thus making the risk of miscarriage a moot point. After research, I decided not to imperil the life of this unborn child and opted to wait to have the amniocentesis until my baby could be safely delivered in the event of any problems.

I did, however, have the ultrasound tests periodically. They helped to reassure me, in that the measurements of the leg bones were always within the normal range. In fact, there seemed to be nothing unusual at all in the tests. And they indicated that the baby was a boy. The family named him Aiden, a celtic name that means "little fiery one." At 7 months, the amniocentesis was performed. Afterward, I rested in bed, reading and cross-stitching. I considered the options facing us in the event that Aiden had Down's Syndrome: we could raise an impaired child, giving our all to be sure he had every chance at a full and productive life. I knew that abortion would be an option offered. I was told the procedure could save me some of the heartache of the years ahead. But it would also destroy any chance of the wonder and joy of raising a special child. Finally, I decided to find out all I could about the syndrome in order to give Aiden every possible option for a happy life.

Within days I received the results of the amniocentesis: no Down's Syndrome. My relief was almost tangible. I happily began preparations for a "normal" baby. On 24 July 1997, my doctor induced pregnancy because my little boy was getting quite large. With two friends and my husband present, I began the birthing process. I labored from 7:00 A.M. until 3:16 in the afternoon, when Aiden made his appearance. I knew something was wrong immediately. As Aiden's head emerged, I saw an odd bump in the middle of his face. As I caught a glimpse of his profile, I thought the bump looked like a tiny duck's bill. The nurses began moving briskly about the room. They swept the baby away before I was able to see him clearly. The atmosphere in the room abruptly changed. Everyone became serious, almost grim. They barked curt orders to each other. No one would meet my eyes.

I'd had an impression of a gaping black hole and two startled dark eyes. Then the nurses had taken the baby across the room, placing him on a raised stand. They closed in around him, obscuring my view. "What's wrong?" I repeatedly asked. "Is my baby okay?" No one answered me as nurses moved in and out of the room. I looked to my obstetrician. "We have a little cleft here." He didn't meet my eyes, but turned away toward my son. Cleft. I had a vague idea of a cleft being some sort of mouth problem. I knew that a cleft in a rock was a split. It dawned on me suddenly: a split mouth. The ugly word *harelip* flitted through my mind. My heart raced as I awaited word of my child. One of my girlfriends grabbed my hand and began to pray aloud. I felt calmed, ready to face this crisis.

After several minutes, a young nurse approached my bedside with a small white bundle. She placed Aiden in my arms and stepped away. Looking down into the face of my son, I immediately saw a distorted nose, with both nostrils distended outward and no philtral lines. The tip of Aiden's nose was growing from his lip. There was no barrier of flesh between his nostrils. Each nostril was open completely into the mouth cavity. Further inspection revealed that there was no roof in Aiden's mouth. He had gums on each side and a little piece of gum in the center of the front of his mouth. This piece has been pushed outward as he had grown; it was the little "duckbill" that I had seen. Aiden's father quietly stepped out of the room.

I felt indescribable sorrow and a twisting pain like a knife in my heart. Then I lifted my gaze to see two calm eyes staring intently into my own. The shock of seeing Aiden's face was suddenly dimmed by an overwhelming love and protectiveness. This was my son, my precious child. I was going to do anything it took to make sure he was okay. I began peppering the nurses with questions: "How can we help him?" "Can he eat?" "Can this be fixed?" Unfortunately, no one had answers. Eventually, the doctor left to see other expectant mothers, and the nurses continued their work on the maternity wing.

My husband returned. It was obvious he had been crying. He told me he had called his parents to tell them about our son. We began to plan how to break the news to the four little children at home waiting excitedly for word about their new baby brother. We borrowed a Polaroid camera from the nurse's station and took a picture of Aiden for his father to take home. We decided he would show it to the children before they came to meet their baby brother. We thought it would help take the shock out of seeing his little disfigured face. We would tell them that Aiden had a "broken lip" and the doctors would fix it over time. Aiden's father went home to prepare the other children for the sight of their new brother.

Within a couple of hours I had been left alone in the room with my child. I rocked him and sang. I didn't cry, but a single tear coursed my cheek. After some time had passed, a pretty nurse entered the room with some printed information on cleft palates.

Most of it was of little use because of the severity of Aiden's cleft presentation, but it did contain the address and phone number of the Cleft Palate Foundation. I dialed the phone, anxious to find any information on how to help my son. A cheery voice answered, explaining several basic facts about clefting and taking down our address in order to send more information. It would arrive in approximately 5 days. Five days! I grew angry at the fact that no one at the hospital had given me clear answers to my questions about my son. I'd learned from the phone call to the Cleft Palate Foundation that clefting occurs in approximately 1 in 700 births. If this was so common, why didn't anyone have any information for me?

I began calling family members to announce the birth of my son, and to explain his disability. A network of people began canvassing the Internet and local libraries to find information. Some called with helpful comments. Some, without realizing it, caused considerable pain. One relative told me that this was my fault, that I obviously didn't eat right during my pregnancy. Another called to tell me that I had this problem because we had a pet rabbit! I stopped answering the telephone. My husband arrived with our four children. Each one looked curiously at the baby with his "broken lip," then promptly ignored him as they became fascinated with the moveable bed. In their simple way, they accepted Aiden as he was, with the knowledge that he would one day be "fixed." Other visitors, however, would gasp at the sight of my son's face. I began keeping his face turned away from others until I'd had a chance to describe him. One woman even compared Aiden's face to that of the Disney cartoon character Quasimodo in *The Hunchback of Notre Dame*. I learned later with a pang that *Quasimodo* means "semi-formed."

Aiden's pediatrician, Dr. Kurt Heyrman, arrived that evening and told me he was going to set up an appointment for Aiden at the University of Wisconsin Hospitals and Clinics in Madison. He spoke highly of the head of the cleft palate team, Dr. Steven Hardy. Although Madison was over an hour's drive from our home, Dr. Heyrman encouraged us to meet with Dr. Hardy. The

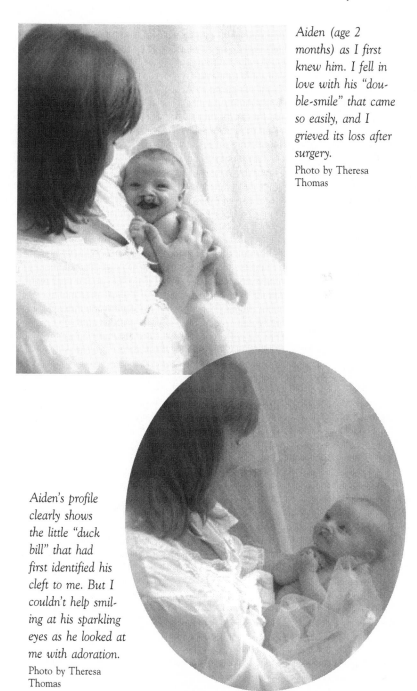

Aiden (age 2 months) as I first knew him. I fell in love with his "double-smile" that came so easily, and I grieved its loss after surgery.
Photo by Theresa Thomas

Aiden's profile clearly shows the little "duck bill" that had first identified his cleft to me. But I couldn't help smiling at his sparkling eyes as he looked at me with adoration.
Photo by Theresa Thomas

appointment would be set up for 2 weeks later. Dr. Heyrman stayed quite a while, answering my questions and working with me to help Aiden learn to eat. His office would also contact the Early Intervention program for our county. A nurse would come to the house and a speech therapist would be assigned to work with Aiden until he turned 3 years old.

Because Aiden did not have a soft palate, he could not suck. Nursing was out of the question. I began using an electric pump to harvest my milk supply. We tried a number of types of bottles and nipples, including the Ross C.P. Nurser, soft pliant bottles, and the Haberman Feeder. We were told that Aiden would not be released from the hospital until he could eat well. Because Aiden was a big boy—over 9 pounds at birth—he wanted to eat! He lost patience with the slow dripping of the Ross C.P. Nurser. I struggled to feed him only one ounce in an hour's time. Aiden and I both became frustrated. Finally, we found the method that worked for us. The Haberman Feeder consists of a small bottle with a large tube-shaped nipple. In the nipple is a reservoir and filter. The size and pliability of the nipple allowed me to squeeze milk into Aiden's mouth. He feasted hungrily.

After 5 days in the hospital, it looked as though Aiden and I would be able to go home. Needing comfort that Sunday morning, I left Aiden in the arms of a volunteer "cuddler" and attended church service. Several people greeted me with hugs, knowing about my child. During service, the pastor announced Aiden's birth. The congregation applauded. After several announcements were completed, the pastor then asked the church members to pray for my son, explaining his problems with eating, his cleft lip and palate, and our pain. I returned to the hospital feeling stronger and ready to face the challenges ahead. I was told upon my return that Aiden could be released. I called home only to find out that three of our children had the flu. I couldn't take a newborn baby into that house. A friend offered to let us stay at her house for a few days since they were leaving on a trip. I packed up my belongings and my son and moved to my friend's home.

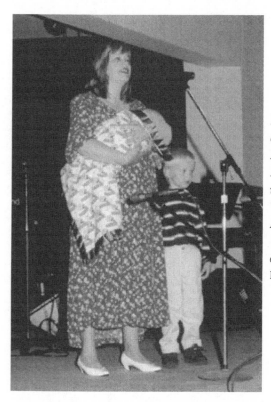

I stood before our church and dedicated Aiden to the Lord just 2 days before his first major surgery. I sang "Be Ye Glad" and Alex, my middle child (age 3), joined me onstage.

Photo by Theresa Thomas

Feeling sad that night, I once again bundled up my baby and headed for my church. There was an evening prayer gathering and, being a musician, I knew the music would be a balm to my aching heart. As I arrived, a teenager caught sight of Aiden and backed away, calling him a monster. I covered his face with a blanket. Sitting in the back of the church, with Aiden sleeping in his carrier at my feet, I closed my eyes and wept. Gradually I became aware of a teenage boy kneeling beside my son. Ben and I had known each other since meeting years ago in a theater production. I held my breath as Ben lifted the blanket and gazed into Aiden's face. He lightly smoothed the little fuzzy head with his strong hands. Looking up at me, Ben said softly, "He's beautiful." The heavy weight I'd carried for 5 days fell away completely. We were going to be okay.

I began to educate myself on my son's condition and the potential treatments. I found information on the Internet, in libraries, and through various foundations and associations. Often the information was incomplete and outdated. I interviewed doctors and cleft palate experts. As I gathered this information, I came to realize that there was little out there for young parents to grab onto when faced with the birth of a cleft-affected child. I turned my focus to disseminating information. I published several newspaper and magazine features dealing with clefting in general and my experiences with Aiden. I self-published five hundred copies of a brochure, using pictures of Aiden and filling it with the "first facts" many parents want to know. One article inspired a local hospital to start a foundation named for Aiden to be used in getting these brochures out to hospitals and Early Intervention programs. Since that time, 27,000 of the brochures have been published.

I found myself becoming an advocate for the cleft-affected community at large. I was often called by hospitals in our area to speak with mothers of babies born with a cleft. My name was given out by University of Wisconsin Hospitals to mothers who wanted someone to talk to about their pain and joy upon delivering a special child. I even found myself explaining Aiden's condition to strangers. One afternoon I took Aiden with me to the local grocery store. Once inside, he became fussy, drawing the attention of several people. Most adults would glance at him, gasp, and let their eyes drop. I became more and more upset at their reactions. "Why don't they just ask me about him?" I wondered. Finally, in the checkout line, a little girl about 7 years old asked me what was wrong with my baby's face. I explained to her in simple terms that his face hadn't finished growing and that we were going to see a doctor who could help finish Aiden's face. As we spoke—she asking questions and me giving answers—a crowd formed. The curious adults who hadn't spoken to me out of fear or politeness gathered around and began asking questions of their own. I began to see a need for the information I had gathered to be made public.

Aiden in recovery. His face is puffy from the fluids given during surgery. He has cotton in his ears where the tubes were placed and tape across his new lip to help keep the stitches in place.

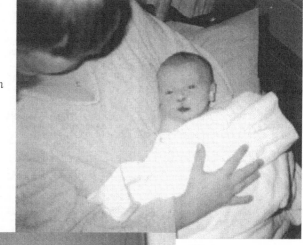

Aiden spent a lot of time watching television or gazing at the photo of his brothers and sisters.

Aiden's first smile with his new lip! It was small and strained, but his cheerful nature was shining through!

Life became a whirl of pumping milk, feeding Aiden, visiting doctors, and writing articles. Church members brought in meals, cleaned our house, and washed our laundry as we learned to cope. At our first appointment with plastic surgeon Steven Hardy, we were impressed by his knowledge and compassion. He refused to leave the room until we were comfortable with his proposals for our child's care. Dr. Hardy mapped out a basic plan, being careful to point out that as a child grows and changes, the plan, too, may change. Aiden would have his first surgery at about 2 months of age. Dr. Hardy would close the clefts in his lip and begin to build a soft palate using tissue inside of Aiden's mouth. An ENT would insert tubes in Aiden's eardrums to aid in drainage. (A child with no soft palate generally does not have fully functioning eustachian tubes, from which chronic ear infections and hearing loss can result.)

Life became easier as we learned how to care for our cheerful little boy. The Early Intervention program assigned speech therapist Heidi Teal to our case. I was delighted to meet her and astounded to find out that this pretty blonde lady had been a classmate of my brother, Ray, and was a member of my church. Every two weeks, and eventually every week, Heidi came to our house and worked with Aiden and me. We began by discussing feeding issues and moved into sound and speech development. Aiden grew to love Heidi, plopping into her lap each visit and giving her hugs and kisses.

Worries continued to plague me as Aiden became less and less responsive to sounds. He was treated for almost continuous ear infections during his first 2 months of life. I began ringing bells to see if he would turn to them. He seldom did. In the week before Aiden's first surgery I began to panic, knowing the little boy I loved so fiercely would return home looking like someone else. I had grown to love his doublewide smile and little, flat nose. This was the face of the child I knew and adored. What would happen when he changed? Would I know him? Would he still be Aiden? What if I didn't recognize my own child? I engaged a photographer to take a series of pictures of Aiden and me. She cap-

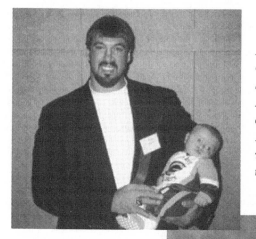

Aiden with Blaise Winter who had become a friend and gave encouragement. Aiden donned his Packer outfit for the day. Notice Blaise's Superbowl ring—Aiden kept trying to grab and eat it!

Showing off his beautiful new lip!
Photo by Theresa Thomas

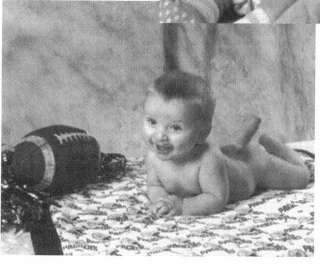

A Packer fan to the skin!
Photo by Theresa Thomas

tured the precious double smiles and his beautiful face. I vowed to have copies of these pictures made to give to Aiden when he was older in order to show him how much I loved him—just as he was!

The surgery was on a brisk October day. We left the children in the care of relatives and traveled to Madison. Aiden couldn't be fed prior to surgery, and he became a little cranky while waiting. Dr. Hardy, the ENT, an anesthesiologist, and several nurses went over the procedures and answered our questions. We changed Aiden into some blue hospital pajamas and handed him to a nurse. We were escorted to the surgical waiting area. Five interminable hours passed as we stared at magazine pages without seeing the words. Finally, Dr. Hardy arrived. Smiling, he told us Aiden had done very well. The tubes were in place, his lip was closed, and most of a soft palate had been constructed.

We were escorted to the recovery room, where I could hold Aiden in a rocking chair. He was a bit dusky in color so the nurses had an oxygen tube blowing across his face. He was puffy from the fluids used in the surgery and his face had great smears of blood. Two angry lines of stitches ran down his upper lip... but he had an upper lip! His nose looked more normal. His arms were encased in "no-no's"—stiff, cloth-covered guards that kept his hands away from his stitches. They were decorated with blue L shapes and little pink bows—L-bows, to keep his elbows from bending. When he finally opened his eyes, I recognized him! My apprehension dissolved. He was still my precious boy.

He was moved to the pediatric intensive care unit (PICU) for observation. This is typical when a child has surgery, especially in his mouth or throat. We were told that if Aiden's throat or mouth began to swell, the nurses in the PICU would be able to take care of the problem. I watched the other parents on the floor. They moved as though dazed. One mother was carried from the PICU when she collapsed after the death of her child. I learned that both her daughters had been killed in a car accident. Aiden would occupy the area vacated by her youngest child. In the next bed, with a curtain drawn around her, was the older

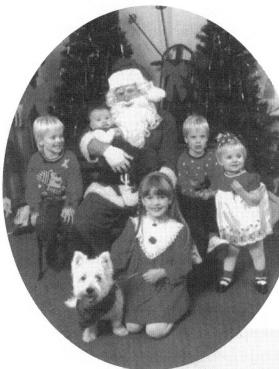

Christmas with the kids. Aiden has healed well and is in preparation for his hard palate surgery that took place 2 months after this photo. (Clockwise from left: Alex, Aiden, Santa, Aaron, Kelsey, Kaitlynne, and Scrubby)

Aiden has a somewhat flattened nose, typical of children with bilateral clefts. Surgery in the future will give him a more normal appearance.

Photo by Theresa Thomas

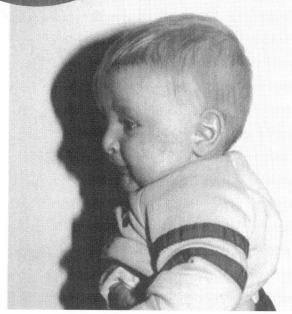

child, who had just died. The grief and pain around me confirmed how fortunate I was to have a child with a problem that could be repaired.

Aiden stayed in the PICU for 26 hours before being moved to a private room. He lay in his bed watching television. Two lines of tape helped to hold his little lip tight. The swelling began to diminish, and the lines didn't look quite so angry. He ate greedily from his Haberman. Three days later, we put Aiden in his car seat for the ride home. He looked at me with his new face and tried to smile. It was difficult and lopsided, but it was his first smile with his new lip. At home, he learned to wriggle out of his "no-no's," and we had to pin them to his sleepers. Eventually, he didn't need them. His return visit to the cleft palate clinic was filled with good news: everything was going just as planned. The next surgery would be when Aiden was 6 months old.

Almost immediately, Aiden's hearing improved. He had literally been hearing the world through liquid—as though under water. The tubes in his ears solved that problem, and his ear infections stopped for good. During the next few months, Aiden was introduced to solid food. He choked and sputtered and grinned. Most of the food leaked out his nose because he didn't have a hard palate yet. Eventually, Aiden learned to push the food further back in his mouth, so that less and less escaped. He learned to sit up, and he learned to manipulate his adoring older brothers and sisters. They helped with therapy exercises and caretaking, running to get diapers or bottles.

On a freezing February day, we made the return trip to Madison for hard palate construction. Again, there was the long wait for the surgery and the time rocking Aiden in the recovery room. Aiden was placed in PICU next to a 2-year-old boy whose parents we had befriended in the surgical waiting area. The little boy had cancer. He did not last the night. Once more I was struck with the blessing of having a healthy little boy. But the visits to Madison for check-ups that followed made me sick to my stomach at the sight and sounds of the hospital. This place of healing was also a place of incredible sorrow.

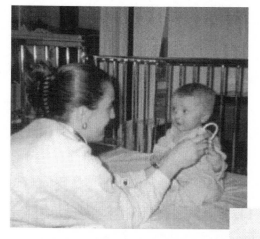

The day of the palate surgery. Aiden (6 months) gets a presurgical check-up.

Mommy and Aiden are ready to walk to the operating room. Aiden is a bit goofy from the medications, keeping me and the nurses in stitches.
Photo by Theresa Thomas

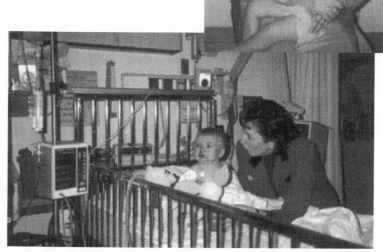

Not a happy baby! Aiden in the Pediatric Intensive Care Unit of University of Wisconsin Hospital. He just wanted to be rocked and cuddled. Here he receives a postoperative check-up.

Aiden was home within 4 days after the hard palate construction. As he began to talk, Heidi became a regular fixture in our home. She worked with Aiden on several sound production problems he was having. She told us she believed he had a high intelligence level, which was in turn causing some problems. Aiden was smart enough to know he was making some sounds incorrectly, but he was also smart enough to develop his own ways to mimic the correct sound—developing some bad habits in the process. Eventually, Aiden developed an "in and out" breathing method of speech: he made certain letter sounds by inhaling rather than exhaling air. We also began to notice that he had trouble with explosive sounds. Aiden began to grow frustrated with his vain attempts at imitating Heidi's speech. At times he would turn his back to her while playing so that he wouldn't have to form the words correctly. His bad habits grew worse. Heidi and I tried to find solutions for his problems, growing frustrated ourselves at times.

Heidi communicated her concerns to the team of doctors in Madison, and Aiden was scheduled for a visit. A *nasopharyngoscope*, a telescopic instrument inserted in the nose, was used to examine the back of Aiden's throat. It was found that his soft palate did not have enough tissue to effectively close when he pronounced certain consonants. The ENTs, audiologists, speech therapists, and Dr. Hardy agreed that another surgery was necessary to improve Aiden's speech function. He had just turned 2 when we made the trip for his third surgery. Dr. Hardy performed a modified pharyngoplasty, closing most of the opening between the soft palate and the throat.

This time, when we arrived in recovery, Dr. Hardy told us that Aiden had had some problems. My heart raced as I heard him telling us that Aiden had stopped breathing twice in recovery and had had to be resuscitated. I looked at my child sleeping in the bed. We could have lost him. Two different theories have emerged as to the cause of Aiden's problems after the operation. One theory, probably a bit more accurate, is that the anesthetic administered caused Aiden to relax to the point of not

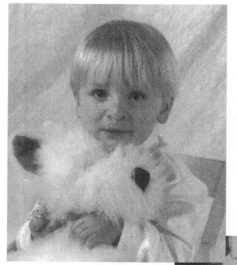

A charmer with the most beautiful eyes. It was those eyes that drew me in and made me fall in love. Slight scarring is visible on his lip around his nostrils. This will change as he undergoes rhinoplasy.
Photo by Theresa Thomas

Clowning in his high chair. Two-year-old Aiden still shows some misshaping of the nose and flattened nostrils, but his lip has gained more flexibility as he has aged.

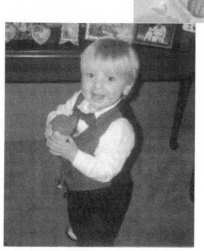

Aiden bounces back quickly to his happy-go-lucky self. Here he is all "duded-up" for a visit to Grandma and Grandpa's house.

breathing during recovery. Another theory, of which there was no evidence, is that his vocal cords may have been nicked, causing them to snap shut.

Only days before the surgery I had attended the funeral of Jan Lenz, a woman who had been like a second mother to me. The grief, compounded with my fear of losing Aiden, brought me to tears. Aiden was given a private room without having to go to the PICU again. It was a small mercy and a great relief—no more roommates who could die in the night. I used the time while Aiden slept in this private room to write the first draft of my first book, A *Special Gift*. The book, published when Aiden was 2 years old, is made up of short, inspirational stories of mothers and their special-needs children. It became a routine for the nurses to tiptoe into the room, check on Aiden, and ask me to read one of the stories to them.

Aiden was a very crabby patient. Not knowing why he hurt so badly, he refused to eat. The only time he was comforted was when he was in my arms. We spent hours watching videos and rocking in the chair. I was told he could not go home until he could eat. Then, through some mix-up at the hospital, no one delivered his food. I repeatedly asked for his meals, was repeatedly told they would be delivered, and grew frustrated as 2 days passed. I sent visitors out for yogurt and bananas. After 4 days, Aiden finally ate a few bites of yogurt and a bite of banana. He was proclaimed "fine" by the attending physician and sent home. We never did get a meal from the hospital during our stay; however, the staff was most apologetic, explaining that a service strike had caused the problem. A few days later we received a formal apology from the hospital.

This recovery was the most difficult of all. Aiden was older now, but not old enough to understand why he was in such pain. He became clingy, wanting to be held all the time. I had just returned to teaching part-time and began feeling guilty about leaving him. We found a caregiver who came to the house. Jenny loved Aiden and all my children, becoming their friend. She learned how to work with Aiden on his speech exercises, even-

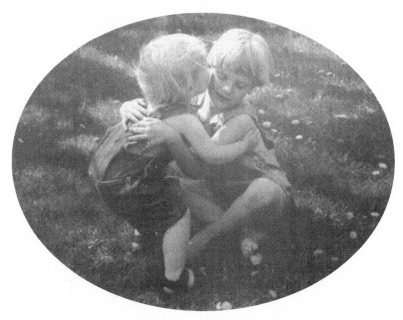

Aiden is always free with his hugs and kisses. (with Aaron)

Enjoying the spring sunshine in the backyard. Aiden and his brothers and sisters have developed a loving relationship. (clockwise from left: Kaitlynne, Aaron, Alex, Kelsey, and Aiden) Photo by Theresa Thomas

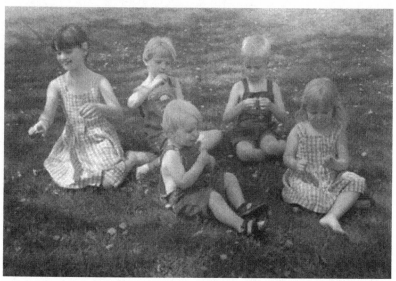

tually driving him to classes as well. In time, Aiden returned to the funny, outgoing little guy he'd always been.

When Aiden turned 3, his relationship with Heidi and Early Intervention ended. He would now receive services from the local school system. As part of the transition, he was given a battery of developmental tests. I knew he would score quite high in intelligence and motor skills—after all, he had been following around his four older siblings for years. Even so, I was surprised by his intelligence ratings: he was performing cognitively as a 6- or 7-year-old! While I didn't expect him to score exceptionally high in speech, I was pleased that his scores had risen from a 4 percent intelligibility level to almost 28 percent in the course of a year.

I knew that Aiden would need some very special care as he moved into the school district. I contacted the teacher of the speech program for 3-year-olds. We discussed Aiden at length, and I asked about his individual speech therapy. I was told that the school did not have individual therapy for children that young; Aiden would be put in a class with other children who had speech issues, some with Down's Syndrome, some with autism. He might get a few minutes of individual attention during class. Fortunately, as an educator, I knew the state of Wisconsin has laws regarding children with special needs. I knew that the school was required to provide the services necessary to my child's individual needs. I began collecting letters and recommendations from Aiden's doctors. All of them stated that he needed extensive individual speech therapy as well as speech and language class.

Once again I was stonewalled, so I contacted an advocate from Madison. She agreed to attend the first individual educational plan meeting with Aiden's teachers. I also contacted the head of the special education program at the school and requested her presence at the meeting, explaining that any special services would have to have her approval before we could proceed. The meeting went well. The advocate explained Wisconsin law clearly and concisely as it applied to Aiden, and Heidi explained Aiden's

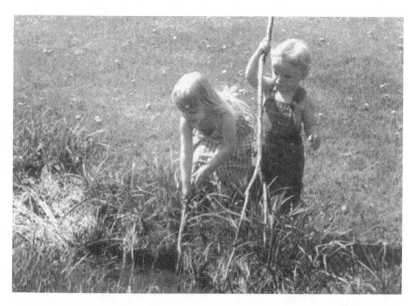

Playing "Huck Finn" is a favorite with the children. Aiden participates in every activity with his brothers and sisters with no restrictions. (Top: Kelsey and Aiden; Bottom, left-to-right: Aiden, Alex, and Aaron)
Photos by Theresa Thomas

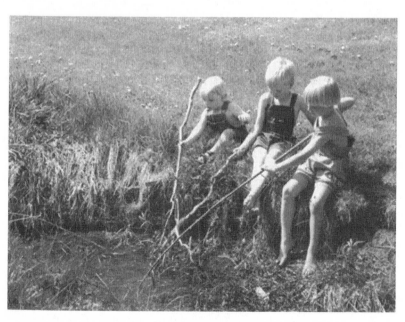

unique needs as a highly intelligent child with a very low level of speech ability. Eventually, it was agreed that Aiden would attend one of the higher cognitive ability groups at one elementary school, and also receive individual speech therapy twice a week at the elementary school that my other children attended. I had taught for a year at that school and knew and liked the speech teacher there, Lynn Goldapske. She became the next stepping stone in Aiden's struggle to speak clearly. Although he missed his Heidi, he grew to love Lynn just as fiercely. They played games and isolated sounds. She sent home worksheets for us to practice at home. His speech became cleaner as he learned to use his mouth and air more effectively.

At about this time, my marriage, already shaky years before, began to unravel. My husband and I agreed to a legal separation in order to explore ways to reach a reconciliation. I have discovered that it is quite common for parents of special-needs children to fall into a pattern of isolation and anger; if the couple involved lack strong communication skills, many of these marriages crumble. Aiden and the other children, although unhappy about the separation, continued to thrive while building strong relationships with both their parents.

Recently, Aiden's main surgeon, Dr. Hardy, announced his departure from the University of Wisconsin Hospitals and Clinics in order to open a practice in Montana. We have begun anew the search for a competent and caring doctor to oversee Aiden's care. We know that he will need to have several more procedures, including bone grafts to build his alveolar ridge (upper gum) and rhinoplasty to help shape his nose. Small challenges continue to pop up periodically. This year we had a 6-month struggle when one of his ear tubes became blocked, was cleared, and became blocked again. He registered a 50 percent hearing loss in that ear and failed a tympanogram, indicating blockage. Finally, after several months and a couple of different types of drops, Aiden is again hearing well. He is making outstanding progress in speech—testing at an intelligibility level of approximately 78 percent.

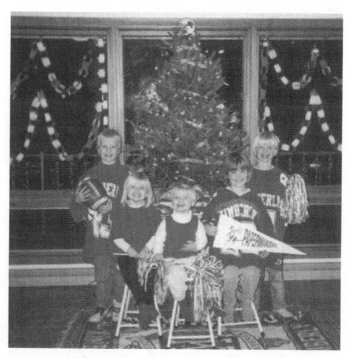

Celebrating Christmas after his third surgery. Aiden's speech improved from a 4 percent intelligibility level to 28 percent and then 78 percent within only a year after surgery! Now he can truly join his siblings as they cheer on our favorite team: the Kimberly High School Papermakers! (Left to right: Alex, Kelsey, Aiden, Kaitlynne, and Aaron)

Aiden is the joy of our family. His bright smile and deep chuckle fill our home and our hearts. We continually swap Aiden stories with friends and relatives. What I would have missed had I never given birth to this wonderful little boy! His passion for life and sense of humor delight everyone who meets him. Four-year-old Aiden and I are frequent guests at meetings of disability awareness groups, Girl Scout troops, and high school classes. We visit new mothers of cleft-affected babies, bringing with us photographs and hope. Aiden enjoys showing people his newest skills. We discuss his birth defect and the progress he has made in overcoming a rough start in life. And we will continue to do so until people begin to understand that a physical defect has nothing whatsoever to do with the worth of a child.

I know that when Aiden is older there will be a time when he asks "Why me?" When that time comes, I will give Aiden a special box I am saving for him. In it, I am collecting cards and letters from families whose lives have been touched by his story through brochures, articles, my books, or a personal visit from him—none of which would exist had I not been gifted with this precious, funny little boy. I do believe that God doesn't make mistakes—Aiden is living proof of that.

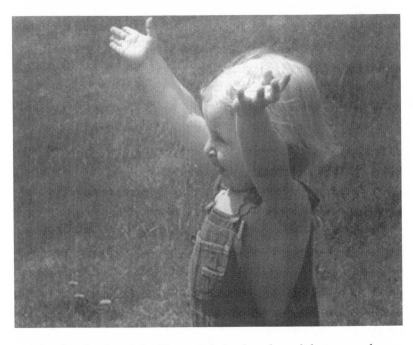

Aiden "catching" sunlight. He certainly has brought sunlight into our family! He has taught us all tolerance, patience, and perseverance. His joyful attitude has been such an example to all of us as we watch him struggle and find success throughout his surgeries and therapies. I wouldn't trade having him for anything in the world! Photo by Theresa Thomas

---

A Model for Introducing a Child with a Cleft Palate into the Elementary Classroom

These pages may be reproduced and shared with your child's teachers, Sunday school class, play groups, and others. You will find that the more other children understand about clefting, the more accepting and supportive they will be with your child.

Opening exercise: Have the children look around the room at each other. Ask them to point out the differences amongst themselves. Begin with such things as hair color, height, and gender. Point out that even children with the "same color" hair or skin do not have *exactly* the same hair or skin color.

Diversity statement: "Boys and girls, we can see that every person in this room is very special. No one is exactly the same as anyone else. What do you think the world would be like if everyone was exactly the same?"

Discussion: Focus on how boring the world would be. Ask the children to discuss who would perform different tasks if we all had the same talents and abilities.

Refocus: "Sometimes our differences are things we are born with, such as our hair or eye color. Sometimes our differences are things we learn, such as being able to play football or to play an instrument. Sometimes our differences can help others. Sometimes we need help with our differences." Begin discussing how we can help others or how we may have seen others being helped: for example, we may have seen a blind person being guided by a trained dog. We may have seen a tall lady reach something on a high shelf for someone not as tall. We may have seen a child use a wheelchair to move about a room.

Diversity statement: "Sometimes a baby is born with a difference or a disability." Discuss the meaning of *disability*, citing examples of various disabilities. Point out that not every disability affects the ability of the brain. For example, a child who uses a wheelchair or a child who cannot hear is not any less intelligent than other children because of these things.

Discussion: "Do you know anyone with a disability? How is that person the same as you? How is he or she different?"

Refocus: "Today we would like to discuss one type of difference called a *cleft lip* or *palate*." When a baby begins growing, the face comes together from the sides. It meets up in the middle, right under the nose. Put your finger on the area under your nose. Do you feel a little dent and two raised lines? That is where your face finished forming. Now feel the roof of your mouth with your tongue. Do you feel a long ridge running from the front of your mouth to the back? That is where the roof of your mouth finished forming. Sometimes a baby's mouth does not finish growing. When that happens, there is a gap or opening called a *cleft*. A cleft does not hurt the baby. Sometimes a cleft is only in the lip area or on the roof of the mouth. Sometimes it is in both places. A cleft can be on one side or on both sides.

"When a baby is born with a cleft, the parents take the baby to a doctor. The doctor performs surgery to close up the cleft and help the baby's mouth finish growing. Sometimes the doctor has to perform more than one surgery. After surgery, some children have to learn to speak clearly. They may not be able to say some of the letter sounds without practicing with a special teacher

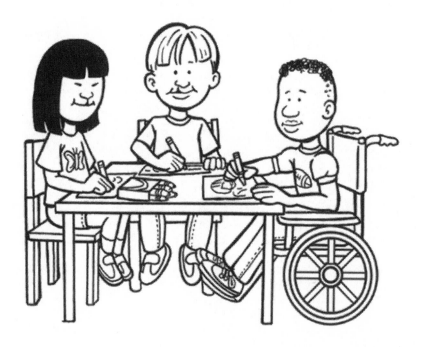

called a *speech therapist*. The speech therapist helps the child learn to speak clearly. For some children, learning to speak clearly may take a long time. It may not take a long time for others. When a child cannot speak clearly because of a cleft, it does not mean that the child is not as intelligent as other children. It just means that he or she has to get used to the changes the doctor made in his or her mouth. Being born with a cleft is just like any other type of difference. And remember, we saw that every child is different and special."

At this point the cleft-affected child can be introduced. Begin by having her tell about herself, including such things as family members, pets, hobbies, and interests. The other children may see that they have some of the same interests as she does. If the child is not shy, have her point out any surgical marks and explain how they were formed. Allow the child to share "before" and "after" pictures with the class. The child and her parent or guardian might be willing to answer questions from the other children in the class. If there are any special considerations that should be made in the classroom, explain them to the children. For example, if the child uses some sign language, explain this to the children and teach them some simple signs. Let the children know that the cleft-affected child may leave the classroom once or twice a week to work with the speech therapist.

Emphasize that, although there are some differences in her speech or looks, this child is just the same as any other child in the class. Celebrate diversity! Once the introductory session is completed, treat the cleft-affected child as you would any other child in the classroom. Keep a watchful eye out for any teasing and nip it in the bud. Encourage the cleft-affected child to participate fully in all activities. Always remember that she is a child first and cleft-affected second.

Additional Resources

Cleft-Related Resources

AboutFace
PO Box 458
Crystal Lake IL 60039

(888) 486-1209
www.aboutfaceusa.org

American Academy of Facial Plastic and Reconstructive Surgery
1110 Vermont Ave., NW
Washington DC 20005

American Cleft Palate Association
104 S. Estes Dr., Suite 204
Chapel Hill NC 27514
E-mail: cleftline@AOL.com

(800) 24-CLEFT
www.cleftline.org

The American Society of Plastic and Reconstructive Surgeons
444 East Algonquin Rd.
Arlington Heights IL 60005
www.plasticsurgery.org

American Speech-Language-Hearing Association
10801 Rockville Pike
Rockville MD 20852

The Center for Craniofacial Anomalies, University of Illinois at Chicago
PO Box 6998, Room 476
CME M/C 588
Chicago IL 60680

The Children's Craniofacial Association
12200 Park Central Dr., Suite 180   (972) 566-5980
Dallas TX 75251   www.ccakids.com

Children's Defense Fund
25 East St., NW
Washington DC 20001

Early Education Intervention Network
26 S. Main St., #287   (603) 228-2040
Concord NH 03301   www.eein.org

FACES (a nonprofit organization serving children and adults throughout the United States with severe craniofacial deformities resulting from birth defects, injuries, or disease)
PO Box 11082
Chattanooga TN 37401

Forward Face, Institute of Reconstructive Plastic Surgery
NYU Medical Center
560 1st Ave.
New York NY 10016

Foundation for Faces of Children
PO Box 1361
Brookline MA 02146

Health Insurance Association of America
1001 Pennsylvania Ave., NW
Washington DC 20004

The Hospital for Sick Children, Cleft Lip and Palate Program
555 University Ave.
Toronto, Ontario M5G 1X8
Canada

La Leche League International (an organization whose sole purpose is helping breastfeeding mothers)
9616 Minneapolis Ave.
Franklin Park IL 60131

Medical Missions Foundation
http://members.tripod.com/~medical missions/mmf/mmf.html

National Association for the Education of Young Children
1509 16th St., NW
Washington DC 20036-1426

National Association of Insurance Commissioners
120 W. 12th St., Suite 1100
Kansas City MO 64105

National Association of State Directors of Special Education
1800 Diagonal Rd., Suite 320
Alexandria VA 22314

National Center for Clinical Infant Programs
2000 14th St. N., Suite 380
Arlington VA 22201-2500

National Health Information Center
PO Box 1133
Washington DC 20013

The New Face Foundation (a nonprofit organization that treats children born with facial and craniofacial deformities)
www.newfacefoundation.com

Northwestern University Cleft Lip and Palate Institute (Chicago)
www.nuds.nwu.edu/clphome.htm

Mead Johnson (a manufacturer of bottles and other infant products)
(812) 429-6321

Medela, Inc. (a manufacturer of bottles and other infant products)
PO Box 660
McHenry IL 60051   (800) 435-8316

PACER Center (Advocacy center that helps parents understand education laws and helps them obtain a proper education for their children)
4826 Chicago Ave. S.
Minneapolis MN 55417

Tennessee Craniofacial Center
T.C. Thompson Children's Hospital
975 E. Third St.
Chattanooga TN 37403
Wide Smiles
www.widesmiles.org   widesmiles@aol.com

General Resources

Check your local library or the Internet for phone numbers or addresses for the following organizations in your state. Each state's organizations may work in a slightly different manner; check with each group for individual programs.

Bureau of Public Health: Programs for children with special health care needs

Department of Public Instruction: Programs and educational rights for children with disabilities

Insurance Commissioner: Information about or problems with insurance

Birth to Three or Early Intervention Office: Information about early childhood intervention; you may also contact these offices on a local level via hospitals in your area or listings in the telephone directory.

Local hospitals, clinics, or referral services: Information about craniofacial or cleft palate teams in your state; you may also wish to contact the larger hospitals in your state.

Partial Guide to Clinics/Teams by State

This listing is incomplete and does not serve as an endorsement of any of the listed clinics. These may also serve as a contact point for additional information or a listing of clinics in your area. The American Cleft Palate Association and the Wide Smiles website have extensive listings of teams and physicians in each state.

Alabama

Birmingham Cleft Lip and Palate Team
1616 6th Ave.
South Birmingham AL 35233

Montgomery Cleft Palate Team
2127 S.E. Blvd.
Montgomery AL 36199

Arkansas

Arkansas Children's Hospital
800 Marshal St.
Little Rock AR 72202

California

Cedars Sinai Medical Center—Cleft Palate Clinic
444 South Sam Vincente Blvd.
Los Angeles CA 90048

Central California Oral & Maxiofacial Surgical Group
1111 E. Herndon #119
Fresno CA 93720

Children's Hospital, Oakland—Craniofacial Surgery
747 52nd St.
Oakland CA 94609

Craniofacial Center
UCSF S-747 Medical Science Building
513 Parnassus Ave.
San Francisco CA 94143

Encino Cleft Palate Clinic
16633 Ventura Blvd., Suite 110
Encino CA 91436   (818) 981-3333

Eureka Cleft Palate Clinic
2121 Myrtle Ave.
Eureka CA 95501   (707) 442-6463

Fresno Cleft Palate Clinic
3151 North Millbrook
Fresno CA 93703   (209) 255-3000

Kaweah Cleft Palate Clinic
400 West Mineral King
Visalia CA 93291

Loma Linda University
11370 Anderson
Loma Linda CA 92354

Long Beach Medical Center—Cleft Palate Clinic
2801 Atlantic Ave.
Long Beach CA 90801

Pleasant Hill Cleft Palate Clinic
490 Golf Club Rd.
Pleasant Hill CA 94523

San Jose Cleft Palate Clinic
2516 Samaritan Dr., Suite H
San Jose CA 95124

San Joaquin General Hospital
PO Box 1020
Stockton CA 95207

UCLA Harbor General Hospital
100 West Carson St.
Box 25
Torrance CA 90509

Colorado

Cleft Palate Clinic, Children's Hospital
1056 East 19th Ave.
Denver CO 80218

Colorado SPR Penrose Hospital
2215 North Cascade Ave.
Colorado Springs CO 80933

Rose Medical Center
4567 E. Ninth Ave.
Denver CO 80220

Connecticut

Newington Children's Hospital
181 East Cedar St.
Newington CT 06111-1540

Yale Craniofacial Center
PO Box 208041
333 Cedar St.
New Haven CT 06520

Delaware

Medical Center of Delaware
PO Box 6001
Newark DE 19718

Florida

Florida USF Referral Center
Florida Cleft Palate Clinic
1 Davis Blvd., Suite 502
Tampa FL 33606

Tampa Bay Craniofacial Center
801 West Martin Luther King Blvd.
Tampa FL 33603

University Medical, Cleft Palate Clinic
655 West 8th St.
Jacksonville FL 32209

University of Miami, Division of Plastic Surgery
PO Box 16960
Jacksonville FL 33101

University of Miami School of Medicine
6601 Southwest 80th St., Suite 112
Miami FL 33143

Winter Park Cleft Palate Clinic
132 Benmore Dr.
Winter Park FL 32792

Georgia

Emory University for Cleft and Craniofacial Anomalies
1365 Clifton Rd. NE
Atlanta GA 30322

Scottish Rite Cleft Palate Clinic
5455 Meridian Mark Rd., Suite 200
Atlanta GA 30342

Atlanta Cleft Palate Clinic
975 Johnson Ferry Rd. NE, #500
Atlanta GA 30342

Cleft Palate Clinic
1206 East 66th St.
Savannah GA 31404

Hawaii

Straub Clinic and Hospital
888 S. King St.
Honolulu HI 96813

Illinois

Chicago Cleft Palate Clinic, Division of Plastic Surgery
Chicago Cook County Hospital
1835 W. Harrison St.
Chicago IL 60612

Chicago Children's Memorial Hospital
2300 Children's Plaza
Chicago IL 60614

Craniofacial Center at Chicago
808 S. Wood
Chicago IL 60612

Peoria Cleft Palate Clinic
900 Main St., Suite 500
Peoria IL 61602

Rock Island Cleft Palate Clinic
Augusta College
Rock Island IL 61201

Urbana Cleft Palate Clinic
602 W. University Ave.
Urbana IL 61901

Indiana

Indianapolis Cleft Palate Clinic
7439 Woodland Dr.
Indianapolis IN 46278

Riley Hospital Craniofacial Team
702 Barnhill Dr., Room 2514
Indianapolis IN 46202

Iowa

Cedar Rapids Cleft Palate Clinic
3705 River Ridge Dr. NE
Cedar Rapids IA 52402

University of Iowa Craniofacial Team
University of Iowa Hospitals and Clinics
Iowa City IA 52246

Kansas

Plastic and Reconstructive Surgery Center
College Medical Building, Suite 204
5520 College Blvd.
Overland Park KS 66211

Wichita Surgery Center
825 North Hillside
Wichita KS 67214

Louisiana

Cleft Palate Clinic, Children's Hospital
200 Henry Clay Ave.
New Orleans LA 70118

New Orleans Cleft Palate Clinic
1514 Jefferson Hwy.
New Orleans LA 70121

Sidell Cleft Palate Clinic
1015 Florida Ave.
Sidell LA 70458

Maine

Augusta Children with Special Health Needs
151 Capitol St.
Augusta ME 04333

Southfield Cleft Palate Clinic
16001 W. Nine Mile Rd., 3rd Floor Fisher Center
Southfield ME 48075

Maryland

Kernan Hospital
2200 Kernan Dr.
Baltimore MD 21207

Craniofacial Center
601 North Caroline McElderry 8
Baltimore MD 21287

Craniofacial Center, University of Maryland
419 West Redwood St.
Baltimore MD 21201

Massachusetts

Boston New England Medical Center
755 Washington St.
Boston MA 02111

Children's Hospital
300 Longwood Ave.
Boston MA 02115

Michigan

University of Michigan Hospital
1500 East Medical Center
Ann Arbor MI 48109

Henry Ford Hospital
2799 West Grand Blvd.
Detroit MI 48202

Cleft Palate Clinic, Blodgett Hospital
1840 Wealthy SE

Grand Rapids MI 49506

Sparrow Hospital
7 Foster
PO Box 30480
Lansing MI 48909

Minnesota

Mayo Clinic
200 First St. SW
Rochester MN 55905

Missouri

Mid-America Cleft and Craniofacial Program
St. Luke's Health Care System
4400 Wornall Rd.
Kansas City MO 64111

Nebraska

Lincoln Cleft Palate Clinic
857 South 48th St.
Lincoln NE 68510

Omaha Cleft Palate Clinic
555 North 30th St.
Omaha NE 68154

New Jersey

Cleft Palate Clinic
684 Broadway
Paterson NJ 07042

Newark University Hospital, Division of Plastic Surgery
100 Bergen St.
Newark NJ 07103

The Regional Cleft Palate Center, Monmouth Medical Center
300 2nd Ave.
Long Branch NJ 07726

St. Joseph's Hospital, Craniofacial
703 Main St.
Paterson NJ 07503

New Mexico

New Mexico Cleft Palate Institute
801 Encino Pl., NE
Albuquerque NM 87102

New York

Craniofacial Disorders Clinic
111 East 210th St.
Bronx NY 10467

University Hospital at Stony Brook
33 Research Way
East Setauket NY 11733

Long Island Jewish Medical Center, Craniofacial Disorders
New Hyde Park NY 11042

St. Charles Hospital
220 Belle Terre Rd.
Port Jefferson NY 11777

North Carolina

University of North Carolina Craniofacial
Chapel Hill NC 27599

Durham Cleft Palate Team
Box 3974
Durham NC 27710

Moses Cone Memorial Hospital
Greensboro NC 27401

Ohio

Oral and Facial Surgery
3040 West Market St.
Akron OH 44333

Children's Hospital
3333 Burnet Ave.
Cincinnati OH 45229

Children's Hospital
Cranio-Facial Clinic
Cleveland OH

University Hospital, Craniofacial Center
11100 Euclid Ave.
Cleveland OH 44106

Columbus Cleft Palate Clinic
1100 Morse Rd.
Columbus OH 43229

Children's Medical Center
1 Children's Plaza
Dayton OH 45404

Youngstown Cleft Palate Clinic
500 Gypsy Ln.
Youngstown OH 44501

Oklahoma

Cleft Palate Clinic, Oklahoma Children's Memorial Hospital
940 Northeast 13th St.
Oklahoma City OK 73190

Medical Center of Tulsa
PO Box 35648
Tulsa OK 74135

Oregon

Scott Clinic
9800 Southeast Sunnyside Rd.
Clackamas OR 97015

Child Development and Rehabilitation Center
707 Southwest Gaines Rd.
Portland OR 97201

Pennsylvania

Northwestern Craniofacial Disorders
201 State St.
Erie PA 16507

Cleft Palate Center, Hamot Medical Center
201 State St.
Erie PA 16550

Lancaster Cleft Palate Clinic
223 North Lime St.
Lancaster PA 17602

St. Christopher Hospital, Cleft Palate Center
Front and Erie
Philadelphia PA 19104

Cleft Palate Center, University of Pittsburgh
317 Salk Hall
Pittsburgh PA 15261

Reading Hospital
Sixth and Spruce
West Reading PA 19602

Williamsport Hospital
420 West 4th St.
Williamsport PA 17701

South Carolina

Trident Regional Medical Center
933 Medical Plaza Dr.
Charleston SC 29406

Medical University of South Carolina, Craniofacial
171 Ashley Ave.
Charleston SC 29425

Roper Hospital
316 Calhoun St.
Charleston SC 29401

Craniofacial Disorders Center
2 Medical Park, Suite 300
Columbia SC 29203

Tennessee

Vanderbilt University Medical Center, Division of Plastic Surgery
2100 Pierce Ave.
Nashville TN 37232

Texas

Children's Hospital of Austin
601 East 15th St.
Austin TX 78701

Corpus Christi Hospital
3533 South Alameda Dr.
Corpus Christi TX 78413

Baylor University Medical Center
3409 Worth St.
Dallas TX 75246

Children's Medical Center of Dallas
1935 Motor St.
Dallas TX 75235

Cleft Palate Clinic
9398 Viscount 1-F
El Paso TX 79925

Cleft Palate–Craniofacial Team
6516 John Freeman Ave.
Houston TX 77030

Texas Tech University, Cleft Palate Team
3601 Fourth Ave.
Lubbock TX 79430

Cleft Palate and Craniofacial Team
South West Texas Methodist Hospital
7700 Floyd Curl Dr.
San Antonio TX 78229

Utah

Primary Children's Medical Center, Craniofacial and Plastic Surgery
100 North Medical Dr.
Salt Lake City UT 84113

Virginia

Fairfax Hospital Center for Facial Rehabilitation
3300 Gallows Rd.
Fall Church VA 22046

Children's Craniofacial Center
601 Children's Ln.
Norfolk VA 23507

MCV Hospital—Facial Rehabilitation Center
PO Box 980154
Richmond VA 23298

Medical College of Virginia, Center for Facial Reconstruction
Box 154
Richmond VA 23298

Washington

Children's Hospital and Medical Center, Craniofacial Team
4800 Sand Point Way, NE
Seattle WA 98105

Cleft Palate Clinic
3629 South D St.
Tacoma WA 98408

West Virginia

West Virginia University
Morgantown WV 26506

Washington, DC

DC General Hospital
19th and Massachusetts
Washington DC 20003

Georgetown University Medical Center, Craniofacial Team
3800 Reservoir Rd. NW
Washington DC 20607

Children's National Medical Center
111 Michigan Ave. NW
Washington DC 20010

Wisconsin

University of Wisconsin Hospital and Clinics, Cleft Palate Team
600 North Highland
Madison WI 53792

Children's Hospital of Milwaukee
9000 West Wisconsin Ave.
Milwaukee WI 53226

APPENDIX C

How to Form a Support Group

Before deciding to form a support group, check to see if one already exists in your area. This may be done by contacting the Cleft Palate Association (see Appendix B: Additional Resources), your local hospital, or the cleft palate team closest to your area. If there is no support group in your area, starting one can be a rewarding and enriching undertaking. Not only will you be providing a needed service to other parents in your situation, but also you will find strength in talking with people who truly understand what you may be going through. There are several steps in forming a group. If you are working with another parent, go over these steps together.

Step 1: Decide on the type of support group you wish to form. Will your group include only parents of cleft-affected children? Will it include parents of children with other craniofacial disorders, speech disorders, any type of disorder? Will your group have a secular or spiritual basis? Will your group be for mothers, fathers, or both? Will your group be adults only or will you have playgroups for the children? Will teenagers or young adults who were born with clefts be invited to join? Decide on the purpose of the group. Will you be a social group? Will you sponsor speakers or activities? Will you host educational sessions?

Step 2: Find a place and time to meet, and decide how long each meeting will last (1½ to 2 hours is a good length of time for a meeting and can include socializing after the meeting). Decide how often the group will meet. Once a week, once a month, once every other month? Many churches make available their recreational spaces for nonprofit groups and support groups. These groups may or may not be church affiliated. Contact local schools and community centers. Many will waive their fee once the purpose of the group is understood. Some have minimal fees for custodial services. Small groups may meet in houses. One person may volunteer to host all the meetings, or you may rotate houses.

Step 3: Will your group charge a meeting fee (to cover costs) or provide childcare? Contact local high schools and middle schools for a list of young people who may provide baby-sitting. If you are providing childcare for special-needs children, some training may be necessary. You might require that each person in the group take a turn baby-sitting at a meeting.

Step 4: Recruit members by making up posters or flyers. A computer-generated information sheet is fine. You may want to add a graphic or a picture of a child with a cleft lip. Be sure to mention that this is an invitation to be a part of a new support group. State the type of group, the meeting time, the meeting place, costs, and who is invited to join.

Step 5: Distribute your information at any of the following locations: Birth to Three centers, Early Childhood centers, daycares, YMCAs, parenting groups, parenting websites, bulletin boards in public areas, local hospitals and clinics, newsletters. Run a few ads in the local newspaper. Ask the paper if they run this sort of ad free for nonprofit groups, or write a letter to the editor explaining the type of group you are forming, and ask if the charge can be waived. If not, the cost can be covered by any dues or fees collected later.

Step 6: Supply some treats or punch for your first meeting and follow the suggested agenda.

An Agenda for the First Meeting

Call the meeting to order. You might begin by reading a poem, essay, or story that touched you and deals with raising children. Then introduce yourself and give a brief overview of your vision for the group. If the group is small, have each person introduce himself and ask that he share the reason for his interest in the group. If the group is too large for this type of introduction, you could break into smaller groups of up to fifteen and allow time for everyone in the groups to introduce themselves.

After the introductions, you can elect officers or form committees. Suggested committees include: refreshments, publicity and member organization, guest speaker recruitment, crafts or activities, and childcare. Officers should include a president who runs the meetings, a vice president who assists the president, a secretary who records meeting minutes, and a treasurer to handle funds. Each committee should have a chairperson who can help make sure the workload is shared among all members of the group. I recommend that everyone be required to sign up for refreshments on a rotating basis.

You may also wish to include a questionnaire to be filled out on site. Ask about the parents' goals or hopes for the group. Allow space for them to make suggestions for future activities or speakers. The more you allow your members input into the support group, the more successful it will be.

At the first meeting, you may wish to share some of your own stories. It would also be wise to have lined up a couple of other parents who will share their stories. Open the floor and ask anyone else if they would like to share. (Having others prepared to share helps ensure you won't be met with blank stares and silence.) Assure everyone that they will be respected and safe within the support group. However, be prepared to gently guide the topics. You might want to suggest a 5-minute time limit on stories.

Allow time to collect any dues. Have your treasurer open a bank account for the group or collect the money in an envelope for the custodial fees. Adjourn the formal meeting for a social time. Keep your meeting to the time limit promised.

Finding Speakers

Local professionals such as physicians, cleft palate team members, athletes, and educators may be willing to speak to your group. Don't forget those experts who can speak on parenting issues that have nothing to do with clefting. (After all, doesn't every parent need to know about tantrums?) If money is available, you can begin a search for speakers outside of your area who charge a fee. For example, Blaise Winter, former NFL player and motivational speaker (see the Foreword to this book), is available to speak to groups. Fees may be firm or negotiable. Don't be afraid to ask! Contact websites, the Cleft Palate Association, parenting organizations, and other groups for suggestions on speakers.

With any speaker, a contract is critical. The contract should specify the date, time, place, topic, and fee for the speaking engagement. Some speakers also require a certain number of attendees. If you have a high-profile speaker or one who has a broad appeal, advertise with posters or ads to include the general public. Take into consideration a potential increase in audience when deciding on a venue.

Continuing the Support Group

Decide with your board on an evaluation time frame. After a certain number of meetings, have an officers' meeting to decide whether or not the support group is going in the direction you had planned. Be willing to compromise and work toward a unified goal for the group. It may not be exactly what you had originally planned, but is it valuable? Are people finding help and support? If the group is large, you may want to consider breaking up into smaller support groups that meet on a regular basis. These groups could then come together for events such as a visit from a speaker or a trip to a farm or museum for the children. It is critical to remember that *you do not have to do it all yourself.* A good leader is one who can delegate and share authority.

Glossary

This glossary includes terms used by physicians; terms for medical or surgical procedures, equipment, and tests; names of body parts; and other terminology common to clefting. You can use this glossary in conjunction with this book or as an aid to understanding your child's medical condition and team plan for treatment. Not every term in this glossary appears in the text of this book; however, many of the terms will be used in the course of your child's testing and treatment.

Acoustic-Immittance (Tympanometric) Diversity (*see Tympanogram*)

Adenoid—lymphatic tissue located in the back of the throat.

Adhesion—attachment. Lip adhesion is the surgical closure of a lip cleft.

Advocacy—the act of speaking out, working for change or help on behalf of another.

Alimentary Canal—the tract of tubing that runs through the digestion system from the mouth to anus.

Alveolar Ridge—the bony ridge of the maxilla (upper portion of the jaw) and mandible (lower portion of the jaw) which contains the teeth.

Anesthesiologist—a physician who specializes in the administration of drugs to produce sleep and loss of feeling in a patient during surgical procedures.

Anomaly—a change or derivation from what is considered "normal" or typical.

Articulation—the process of forming speech.

Articulation Testing—an assessment during which a specialist gathers information on the formation of speech.

Atresia—the closure or absence of a normal bodily opening.

Audiogram—a graph used to record hearing sensitivity.

Audiologist—a specialist in the science of hearing who has a degree, license, and certification. The audiologist is responsible for testing hearing and diagnosing hearing loss, and will work as a part of the cleft palate team to prevent and/or treat that loss.

Bicuspids—the teeth between the canines (cuspids) and the first molar.

Bridge or Bridge Work—a prosthetic device which replaces missing teeth.

Bilateral—concerning both sides. A bilateral cleft is a double cleft.

Bite—the way the upper and lower teeth are placed in relation to each together (see *occlusion*).

Canine—the pointed teeth between the incisors and bicuspids.

Cardiopulmonary—pertaining to the heart and lungs.

Cineradiography—a film or recording of physical activity, generally used to diagnose velopharyngeal incompetence or insufficiency.

Cognitive—pertaining to intelligence, or conscious knowledge.

Columella—the central, lower tissue part of the nose that separates the nostrils.

Communication Disorder—any situation in which a person is inhibited in his or her ability to express him- or herself and/or understand the communication of others.

Congenital—any deformity or impairment that existed at the time of birth.

Counselor—a person who gives guidance and advice. Generally one trained to guide and aid people in personal or emotional issues.

Complete Cleft—a cleft presentation involving a total split through the palate, gum, or lip.

Craniofacial—of the head and face.

Crossbite—a condition in which the upper teeth are in a placement behind the lower teeth instead of in front of them.

CT Scan—CAT scan involving cross-sectional X rays of the body.

Cuspid—a canine tooth.

Denasality—a quality of speech in which the normal sounds for *m*, *n*, and *ng* are absent (see *hyponasality*).

Dental Arch—the curved placement formed by teeth in correct position.

Dentition (Primary, Mixed, Permanent)—the type, placement, arrangement, and number of teeth. Primary: baby teeth. Mixed: some baby teeth and some permanent teeth. Permanent: adult teeth or second teeth.

Dysfunction—abnormal function.

Eardrum—the tympanic membrane. The eardrum vibrates and transmits sound to the middle ear.

ENT—ear, nose, and throat. The abbreviation commonly used for the specialist working in these areas (see *otolaryngologist*).

Esophagus—the approximately 9-inch tube that runs from the mouth to the diaphragm.

Eustachian Tube—the air duct from the middle ear to the back of the throat. It allows equalization of pressure on both sides of the tympanic membrane (eardrum), and ventilates the middle ear cavity.

Fistula—an opening, such as a hole in the hard palate.

Genetics—the study and science of heredity.

Harelip—a term used by some to indicate a cleft lip. It is considered offensive.

Hearing Impairment—a loss of the ability to hear.

Heredity—characteristics derived from genetic ancestry.

Hypernasality—a greater vocal resonance during speech.

Hyponasality—denasality. A lack of normal vocal resonance during speech. Hyponasality sounds similar to speech during a bad head cold.

Incisor (Central, Lateral)—a tooth used for cutting, generally located at the apex of the mouth.

Incomplete Cleft—a cleft presentation that does not involve a complete split of the palate, gum, or lip.

Interdisciplinary—relating to two or more disciplines working, communicating, or joining together.

Laryngeal—having to do with the larynx.

Larynx—voice box. Contains the vocal cords.

Longitudinal Evaluation—assessment over time.

Malformation—abnormal structure.

Malocclusion—incorrect positioning of the upper teeth in relation to the bottom teeth.

Mandible—the lower portion of the jaw.

Maxilla—the upper jaw.

Microtia—a malformation of the outer ear.

Middle Ear—the portion of the ear behind the eardrum containing three small bones which vibrate to transfer sound to the inner ear.

Maxillofacial—concerning the upper jaw and face.

Molar—back teeth used for grinding food.

Midfacial Retrusion—a condition in which the middle of the face does not grow at the same rate as the rest of the face resulting in a flattened or concave profile.

Myringotomy—a medical procedure in which a small cut is made in the eardrum to allow drainage of fluids.

Nasal Ala—the outer portion of the nostril.

Nasal Emission—emission of air during speech through the nose.

Nasal Regurgitation—expulsion of food or liquids through the nose.

Nasal Tip—the tip of the nose.

Nasoplasty—rhinoplasty. Reconstruction or alteration of the nose.

Neonatal—pertaining to or affecting the newborn infant; the newborn stage, generally the first month after birth.

Nasopharyngoscope—equipment used to examine the back of the throat.

Obturator—a plate that is used to complete closure of the palate, facilitating eating and speaking before reconstructive surgery. It can also be used as a retainer during palate expansion or as a bridge to supply missing teeth.

Occlusion—bite. The placement of the upper teeth in relation to the lower teeth.

Oral Cavity—the mouth.

Orofacial—concerning the mouth and face.

Orthodontics—a specialty concerning proper placement of the teeth and jaws.

Otitis Media—ear infection. An inflammation of the ear with the accumulation of fluids.

Otolaryngologist—ENT. A specialist concerned with treatment and diagnosis of the ear, nose, and throat.

PICU—Pediatric Intensive Care Unit.

Palatal Insufficiency—a lack of tissue of the soft palate resulting in incomplete closure at the back of the throat.

Palate (Soft, Hard)—the roof of the mouth. The hard palate is in the front. The soft palate or *velum* is at the back.

Pediatric Dentistry—a specialist concerned with the care and treatment of children's teeth.

Pediatrician—a specialist concerned with the care and treatment of children.

Pharyngeal Flap—a flap of skin attached to the velum, used to close most of the opening between the velum and the back of the throat.

Pharyngoplasty—a surgical procedure in which a flap of skin is used to connect the soft palate (velum) to the back of the throat to enhance speech production.

Pharynx—the part of the alimentary canal between the mouth and esophagus.

Philtral Lines—the two lines under the nostrils leading to the lip, also known as *prolabium*.

Plastic Surgery—the practice of reconstruction, restoration, and alteration of external defects.

Prelinguistic—before speech.

Premaxilla—the bone of the upper jaw that contains the four front teeth.

Prolabium—philtral lines.

Prosthesis—a man-made device used to replace a missing body part.

Prosthodontist—a specialist concerned with the construction and placement of dental prosthesis devices.

Psychologist—a licensed and/or certified specialist concerned with emotional and mental health.

Psychosocial—relating to the effects of mental and emotional health on social behavior and relationships.

Radiography—X rays.

Resonance—vocal sound concerning the vibration of air through the facial cavities.

Respiratory—concerning the inhaling and exhaling of breath.

Rhinoplasty—reconstruction or alteration of the nose; also known as *nasoplasty*.

Sleep Apnea—brief cessations of breathing during sleep.

Soft Palate—the soft tissue making up the back part of the roof of the mouth, also known as the *velum*.

Speech/Language Pathologist—a licensed and/or certified specialist concerned with the diagnosis and treatment of speech, language, and communication disorders.

Speech Defect—any problem with speech, language, or communication.

Submucous Cleft—a cleft occurring in the muscles under the outer tissue of the soft palate, often diagnosed later than other cleft presentations.

Syndrome—a pattern of anomalies recognized as having a single or specific cause.

Tonsil—lymphoid tissue, two of which are located at the back of the mouth.

Tympanogram—a test that measures pressure on the eardrums and can help detect fluid in the eardrums, blocked tubes, or potential hearing loss.

Unilateral—one-sided. A unilateral cleft occurs on one side of the lip or palate.

Uvula—the small piece of tissue hanging from the soft palate (velum) at the back of the mouth.

Velopharngeal Incompetence/Insufficiency—incomplete closure of the soft palate (velum) with the back of the throat.

Velum—soft palate.

Ventilating Tubes—tubes placed in the eardrum to allow ventilation and drainage, as well as equalization of pressure.

Velopharyngeal Closure—interaction of the muscles of the soft palate and the back of the throat allowing sufficient closure for speech.

Vermilion—lower lip.

Voice—sounds that originate in the larynx.

Zygoma—cheekbone.

Bibliography

Books and Booklets

Allender, Dan B., Ph.D. *The Healing Path: How the Hurts in Your Life Can Lead You to a More Abundant Life.* Colorado Springs, CO: Waterbrook Press, 1999.

Benson, Peter L., Ph.D.; Judy Galbraith, M.A.; and Pamela Espeland. *What Kids Need To Succeed.* Minneapolis, MN: Free Spirit Publishing, Inc., 1994.

Berkowitz, Samuel. *Steps in Habilitation for the Cleft Lip and Palate Child.* Evansville, IN: Mead Johnson & Company, 1979.

Berube, Margery S., Director of Editorial Operations. *The American Heritage Dictionary, Second Edition.* New York: Dell Publishing, 1983.

Bleiberg, Aaron H., and Harry E. Leubling. *Parents' Guide to Cleft Palate Habilitation.* Jericho, NY: Exposition Press, Inc., 1971.

Charkins, Hope, M.S.W. *Children with Facial Difference: A Parents' Guide.* Bethesda, MD: Woodbine House, 1996.

Gruman-Trinkner, Carrie T. *A Special Gift: A Devotional for Mothers of Children with Unique Challenges.* Nashville, TN: Thomas Nelson Publishers, 2000.

Heavilin, Marilyn Willett. *Roses in December.* Eugene, OR: Harvest House Publishers, 1987.

Hickman, Martha Whitmore. *Healing after Loss: Daily Meditations for Working through Grief.* New York: Avon Books, 1994.

Holt, Pat, and Grace Ketterman, M.D. *When You Feel Like Screaming!* Wheaton, IL: Harold Shaw Publishers, 1988.

Hotchner, Tracy. *Pregnancy & Childbirth.* New York: Avon Books, 1984.

Jantz, Gregory L. *Healing the Scars of Emotional Abuse.* Grand Rapids, MI: Fleming H. Revell, A Division of Baker Book House Co., 1995.

La Leche League International. *The Womanly Art of Breastfeeding,* 35th Anniversary Edition. Schaumburg, IL, 1991

Lerner, Harriet Goldhor, Ph.D. *The Dance of Anger.* New York: Harper & Row Publishers, Inc., 1985.

Lewis, Michael B., M.D., and Hermine M. Pashayan, M.D. *Cleft Lip and Palate: Information for the Teenager Born with a Cleft Lip, and/or Cleft Palate.* Pittsburgh, PA: The Cleft Palate Foundation, 1997.

Lipman, Karen S. *Don't Despair Cleft Repair.* Self-Published through Legacy Productions, 1996.

Lynch, Joan I., Ed.D., Chairperson, CPF Publications Committee. *Cleft Lip and Cleft Palate: The First Four Years.* Chapel Hill, NC: Cleft Palate Foundation, 1989.

Lynch, Joan I., Ed.D., Chairperson, CPF Publications Committee. *Feeding an Infant with a Cleft.* Chapel Hill, NC: Cleft Palate Foundation, 1997.

Martin, Frederick N. *Introduction to Audiology.* Englewood Cliffs, NJ: Prentice-Hall, Inc., 1975.

McGuire, Paul. *The Breakthrough Manual.* South Plainfield, NJ: Bridge Publishing, Inc., 1993.

McManus, Margaret A. *Understanding Your Health Insurance Options: A Guide for Families Who Have Children with Special Health Care Needs.* Washington, DC: McManus Health Policy, Inc., 1988.

McWilliams, Betty Jane, Ph.D.; Hughlett L. Morris, Ph.D.; and Ralph L. Shelton, Ph.D. *Cleft Palate Speech.* Burlington, Ontario; Philadelphia, PA: B.C. Decker, Inc., 1984.

Perkins, William H., Ph.D. *Speech Pathology: An Applied Behavioral Science.* Saint Louis, MO: The C. V. Mosby Company, 1971.

Powell, Terry. *Nobody's Perfect.* Wheaton, IL: Victor Books, 1981.

Rosenfeld, Lynn Robinson, L.C.S.W., Ph.D. *Your Child and Health Care.* Baltimore, MD: Paul H. Brookes Publishing Co., 1994.

Siegel, Alice, and Margo McLoone Basta. *The Information Please Kids' Almanac.* New York: Houghton Mifflin Company, 1992.

Smith, Harold Ivan. *A Decembered Grief: Living with Loss while Others Are Celebrating.* Kansas City, MO: Beacon Hill Press, 1999.

Snyder, Gilbert; Samuel Berkowitz; Kenneth R. Bzoch; and Sylvan Stool. *Your Cleft Lip and Palate Child.* Evansville, IN: Mead Johnson & Company.

Tenenbaum, David. *You and Your Medical Debt.* Madison, WI: The Center for Public Representation, Inc.

Van Riper, Charles. *Speech Correction: Principles and Methods.* Englewood Cliffs, NJ: Prentice-Hall, Inc., 1972.

White, James R. *Grieving: Our Path Back to Peace.* Minneapolis, MN: Bethany House Publishers, 1997

Wicka, Donna Konkel, M.A., and Mervyn L. Falk, Ph.D. *Advice to Parents of a Cleft Palate Child.* Springfield, IL: Charles C. Thomas, Publisher, Bannerstone House, 1970.

Winter, Blaise, with William Kushner. *A Reason to Believe.* Coal Valley, IL: Quality Sports Publications, 1998.

Pamphlets, Newsletters, and Articles

ABC for Health. *Advocacy and Benefits Counseling for Families with Children Having Special Health Care Needs.* 1997.

ABLEDATA Database of Assistive Technology. *Funding Assistive Technology.* ABLEDATA Fact Sheet no. 14 (July 1992).

AboutFace, U.S.A. *AboutFace* (informational pamphlet). Limekiln, PA.

AboutFace, U.S.A. *AboutFace* 6, no. 4. (July/August 1992).

American Cleft Palate–Craniofacial Association. "Parameters for the Evaluation and Treatment of Patients with Cleft Lip/Palate or Other Craniofacial Anomalies." *Cleft Palate–Craniofacial Journal* 30, suppl. 1 (1993).

"Breast-feeding the Baby with Special Healthcare Needs: Cleft Lip or Palate and Cystic Fibrosis." *The Exceptional Parent* 29 (November 1999): 52.

Children's Hospital of Wisconsin. Informational Packet. Milwaukee, WI, 1997.

Children's Hospital of Wisconsin. *Practical Advice for Parents.* Milwaukee, WI, 1996.

Cleft Palate Foundation. *For Parents of New-Born Babies With Cleft Lip/Palate.* Pittsburgh, PA, 1989.

Cleft Palate Foundation. *Parents & Patients* 15, no. 4 (November 1991).

Collins, Jane. "Cleft Lip and Palate: Care and Treatment of Child Sufferers." *The Times,* 28 March 2000, sec. 2, p. S15(1). Posted to Health Reference Database.

Danner, S., and E. Cerutti. *Nursing Your Baby with a Cleft Palate or Cleft Lip.* Waco, TX: Childbirth Graphics, 1990.

Department of Health and Social Services, Wisconsin Program for Children with Special Health Care Needs. *Baby Dear, Can You Hear?* Madison, WI, 1992.

Early Intervention Program. *Parent Handbook.* Appleton, WI, 1997.

FACES: The National Association for the Craniofacially Handicapped. *FACES* 10, no. 3 (Christmas 1996).

Greene, Joanne, ed. *Wide Smiles* 2, no. 4 (Spring 1993).

Greene, Joanne, ed. *Wide Smiles* 4, no. 4 (Spring 1994).

Greene, Joanne, ed. *Wide Smiles* 5, no. 1 (Summer 1995).

Greene, Joanne, ed. *Wide Smiles* 5, no. 3 (Winter 1996).

Greene, Joanne, ed. *Wide Smiles* 6, no. 1 (Summer 1996).

Greene, Joanne, ed. *Wide Smiles* 6, no. 4 (Spring 1997).

Greene, Joanne, ed. *Wide Smiles* 6, no. 1 (Summer 1996).

Gruman-Trinkner, Carrie. *Closing the Rift.* Appleton, WI, 1998.

John, Sue Lockett. "Sharing Support." *Focus On the Family with Dr. James Dobson* (January 2001): 10–11.

LaRoi, Heather. "Hand of God." *The* (Appleton, Wis.) *Post Crescent*, 15 April 2000.

Lieff, Susan; Andrew F. Olshan; Martha Werler; Ronald P. Strauss; Joanna Smith; and Allen Mitchell. "Maternal Cigarette Smoking During Pregnancy and Risk of Oral Clefts in Newborns." *American Journal of Epidemiology* 150, 7 (1 October 1999): 683(12).

Martell, Chris. "It's What's Inside That Matters" *Wisconsin State Journal* (Summer 1997).

Mayo Clinic. *Family Health Book, Genetics and Genetic Disorders.* Rochester, MN: Publishing, Inc., 1993.

McCartney, Joan. *When Comments Hurt.* 1993.

MeadJohnson Nutritionals. *Guidelines for Feeding and Care of the Cleft Lip/Palate Infant.* Evansville, IN, 1985.

Medela, Inc. *The Haberman Feeder* (1994).

Milerad, Josef; Ola Larson; Catharina Hagberg; and Margareta Ideberg. "Associated Malformations in Infants with Cleft Lip and Palate: A Prospective, Population-Based Study." *Pediatrics* 100, no. 2 (August 1997): 180.

Mohrbacher, N. *Nursing a Baby with a Cleft Lip or Cleft Palate.* Publication no. 122. Schaumburg, IL: La Leche League International, 1994.

Operation Smile. Informational Packet. Norfolk, VA, 1998.

Outagamie County, WI. *The Early Intervention Program* 17, no. 1 (March 1997).

St. Elizabeth Hospital. Informational Packet. Appleton, WI, 1997.

Trinkner, Carrie. "Faith and Healing." *The* (Appleton, WI) *Post Crescent*, 5 April 1998.

University of Wisconsin Hospital and Clinics. *Health Facts for You: Cleft Palate Repair and Pharyngeal Flap, Home Care Guide.* Madison, WI, 1992.

University of Wisconsin Hospital and Clinics. Informational Packet. 2001.

Vanney, Susan. "Happy Days," *The* (Appleton, Wis.) *Post Crescent,* 22 August 1993.

Warlow, Charles P.; Cathie Sudlow; Steff Lewis; Alison Williams; Jonathan Sandy; and Jonathan Sterne. "Surgeon Experience," letter to the editor. *The Lancet* 355, 9207 (11 March 2000): 932.

West, Ben. "Facing Perfection." *The Guardian* (21 January 1997): T13(1).

Williams, A.C.; J.R. Sandy; S. Thomas; D. Sell; and J.A.C. Sterne. "Influence of Surgeon's Experience on Speech Outcome in Cleft Lip and Palate." *The Lancet* 354, 9191 (13 November 1999): 1697.

Williams, Stephen P. "A New Smoking Peril." *Newsweek* (24 April 2000): 78.

Wisconsin Birth to Three Program. *Parent and Child Rights* (fact sheet). Madison, WI, 1997.

Wisconsin Department of Health & Family Services. *Medical Assistance Coverage for Children With Disabilities or Chronic Illnesses Living at Home.* July 1996.

Wisconsin Department of Health and Social Services, Division of Health. *Healthy Start.* April 1993.

Woon, Maureen. "A Special Gift' Fills a Niche." *The Times* Fox Valley Edition, Appleton, WI (11 May 2000).

Internet Articles/Websites

About Cleft Lip and Cleft Palate. American Cleft Palate-Craniofacial Association. 1997.

Bereavement. BUPA HealthLine. <hcd2.bupa.co.uk/fact-sheets/mosby-factsheets/Bereavement.html> 27 February 2001.

Caring for Your Newborn with Cleft Lip and/or Cleft Palate for Parents, from Parents. Edited by Susan K. MacDonald. <www.samizdat.com/pp2.html> 31 July 1997.

Cheech Marin. <http://www.imdb.com/Name?Cheech+Marin> March 2001.

The Grieving Process Booklet. ADD: Against Drunk Driving. <www.add.ca/grieving.html> January 2001.

Hearing and Behavior in the Child with Cleft Palate. Prescription Parents, Inc. Susan K. MacDonald. <www.samizdat.com/pp4.html> July 1997.

Insurance-Military Links. Wide Smiles. <http://widesmiles.org/military.html> January 2001.

New Parents: Frequently Asked Questions. Wide Smiles.
<www.widesmiles.org> September 2000.

The Orthodontist's Challenge: Treatment of the Patient with Cleft Lip
and Palate. eBody.com, Dr. Donna J. Stenberg.
<www.ebody.com/orthodontics/articles/199908/article27.html>
January 2001.

Parents Helping Parents of Children with Cleft Lip and Palate. Prescription Parents, Inc. <www.samizdat.com/pp1.html> July 1997.

Speech and Language Considerations for the Child with Cleft Palate.
Prescription Parents, Inc. Lenore Daniels Miller, Sc.D., CCC-SLP.
<www.samizdat.com/pp5.html> July 1997.

Speech Following Palatal Surgery. National Institute of Dental and
Craniofacial Research. (ClinicalTrials.gov)
<http://clinicaltrials.gov/ct/gui/c/a1r/action/GetStudy?JServSes-
sionldzone_ct=xwssy05xk1> January 2001.

Wondering Who is Affected by a Cleft? Wide Smiles: Who Has A Cleft?
<www.widesmiles.org/people/who.html> January 2001

WideSmiles Cleft-Links (widesmiles.org)

Arhinia Information by Kristi Branstetter. 1997.

The Big Question: What Makes a Cleft? 1997.

Birth Defect Statistics. 1998. Posted to Cleft-Talk from *Newsweek*,
Spring/Summer 1997; March of Dimes, Perinatal Center, 1997.

Cleft and Fused Fingers/Toes or Fingers Not in Normal Position. 1996.

Cleft Facts. 1996.

Constriction Band Syndrome by Joanne Greene. 1996.

Definition of Stickler Syndrome from The Arthritis Foundations' *Primer
of Rheumatic Diseases.* 1996.

Goldenhar's Syndrome/Boy on Barney. 1996.

Kallmann Syndrome. 1996.

Oral Facial Digital Syndrome Type I. 1997.

Resource—Short Stature and Clefting, Midline Defects. 1996.

Statistics; Increase in Birth Defects 1979–1987 from "A Population-based
Study of the Risk of Recurrence of Birth Defects." *New England
Journal of Medicine* 331, no. 1 (7 July 1994): 1–4.

Vitamin-A Alert. (Credit given to both *Reader's Digest*, March 1996, and
the *New York Times*.) 1996.

Index

U

V

W